The Paradox of Pain: How Memes Make Light of Mental Health Struggles

Pauly

First Printing, 2024

Table of Contents

Page

Chapter 1: Introduction

Suffering is trending. In digital pop culture, memers write "mood," "me," or "same," as an indication of relatability through experiences of misery. Social media users joke about feeling dead inside, going to therapy, and insomnia (for just a few examples, see Thomas, 2017). In the memeworld, a popular trend jokes about depression symptoms in various ways, some openly referring to depression, others more obscurely to "the struggle" (a slang term that designates difficulty in daily living), and any number of other references to mental health. "Depression memes" are not merely memes about depression, but a category of their own, familiar to internet users, who recognize them instantly if they are sufficiently entrenched in internet culture. Depression memes are popular enough that "depression meme" has become a meme in and of itself, as many depression memes refer to depression memes as part of the joke.

Although depression memes describe experiences that correlate to the major symptoms listed in the Diagnostic and Statistical Manual of Mental Disorders (DSM-V) (American Psychological Association, 2013) including, but not limited to: "depressed mood most of the day, nearly every day," "diminished interest or pleasure in all, or almost all, activities," "weight loss…or weight gain," "insomnia or hypersomnia," "fatigue or loss of energy," "feelings of worthlessness," and "thoughts of death" (DSM-V, 2013, p. 160-161), they do not always use them explicitly. Instead, these symptoms become punchlines online in a global litany of jokes that form a universal awareness to suffering through their somewhat casual, ubiquitous rendering of the symptoms in a normalized, glossed-over depiction of individual experience.

As such, I define *suffering* as the tendency of depression memes to use mental health symptoms generically; that is, as universal signs of distress rather than as precise indicators of clinical depression. Via memes, internet users joke about suffering in a highly nuanced online chorus of angst, vaguely aligned with depression symptoms but also more generally referring to the human condition of struggle. Online, users join in the refrain of "mood," contributing to a globalized rhetorical attunement toward suffering. Although some memes refer to specific diagnoses or symptoms, not all do and most take "the struggle" for granted as a part of living on planet Earth. That is, symptom-as-suffering refers to propensity of depression memes to depict human experience as rooted in struggle, rather than happiness. Accordingly, even though I will use the term "depression memes" throughout this book, I approach those memes as speaking not to clinical depression but to the general experience of suffering, as discursively portrayed in parallel to the symptoms of clinical depression. Online, and off, this condition is frequently referred to as "the big sad."

The Big Sad

"The big sad" or "large sad" refers to depression; simultaneously and paradoxically, memes are colloquially referred to as a safeguard against depression (e.g., in the Urban Dictionary definitions discussed above, also see Figure 1.1). Czyzewski (2001) critiqued the 21st century turn of the "current social moods" (p. 268) surrounding the anxieties of post-modernity, tracing a historical path that illustrated the medieval consciousness as comfortable and familiar with violent crime and infectious diseases, whereas the post-modern mind believes them to be growing in intensity and ubiquity during a time when crime and disease are more accurately decreasing (Czyzewski, 2001). The contrast is an interesting one, especially in terms of social "moods" in various time periods. The social moods expressed through depression memes portray the world as collectively suffering, albeit with a focus on the individual sufferer through self-deprecating humor.

Figure 1.1

Memes and The Big Sad

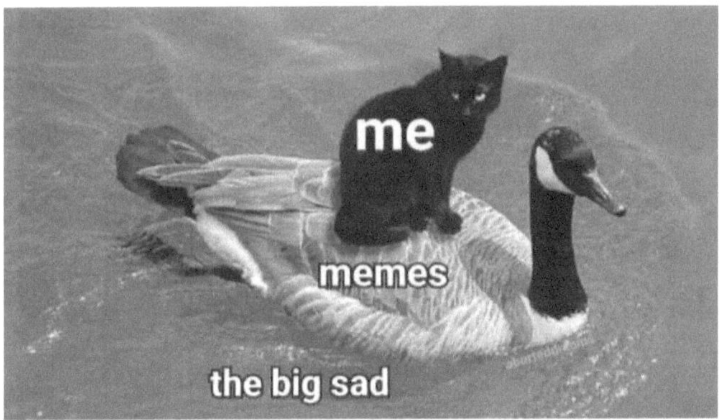

To view memes online is to view the world as in distress, particularly among a certain age group. Teens and twenty-somethings online engage in a collective experience of suffering through memetic practice. Depression memes are internet jokes that utilize an image to make a joke about depression symptoms, diagnoses, experiences, and other related tropes of suffering. Incidentally, in a book on political memes, Huntington

(2017) found that affect was "influential in perceptions of persuasiveness" (p. 164), even if the viewers were not persuaded by the meme itself. Thus, current social moods (as illustrated by memes and otherwise) emerge in and around and on rhetorical environments, mostly without the knowledge or permission of human inhabitants.

Because depression memes have gained some level of virality, they are afforded value in the systems in which they circulate. A meme might be "just a joke," but its circulation and status as a visual enthymeme gives it certain clout in online systems. Some memes are more "relatable" than others, as internet users may choose to comment "same" or "me" on a meme to indicate their agreeance with the premises (explicit and implicit). The trend is not confined to the internet, either—a person conversant in meme culture knows they can verbally use these phrases to another person also familiar with meme culture. As one example, an internet user might comment the word "mood" on an example of suffering, which is expressed in the example from Figure 1.1 (discussed previously), but I have often heard teens and young adults say "mood" aloud when something goes awry. Such is the tendency of memes, even before the internet era; digital platforms merely provide an archivable resource in which to track these trends.

This book is born of experience. One day, as a newly minted PhD student and proud new owner of several chronic conditions, I lay scrolling Pinterest in my habitual attempt to glean a little dopamine out of the chaos. The memes that moved across my screen were filled with sarcasm, irony, and even glee at circumstances that I recognized as symptoms of my own poor mental health. Depression is not the only mental health disorder to receive the meme treatment, either, although I confine myself to it here in the interest of space and specificity; anxiety is almost equally as popular online and is only left out of this book for practical purposes. As meme after meme joked about mental and emotional experiences that, in my experience, were utterly un-funny, I asked myself, "Is everyone depressed?" Of course, that question is neither useful nor answerable, although studies illustrate that rates of depression and suicide increase every year, especially for Millennials and Gen Zs (Curtin & Heron, 2019; Hedegaard, Curtin, & Warner, 2020; Twenge et al., 2010). Instead, I ask, broadly, what do memes say about current discourses of depression?

In the digital atmosphere of today, internet users "breathe" in (by viewing) and "breathe" out (by sharing) particles of cognition and emotion. In an age of worldwide pandemics, polarized politics, environmental malaise, national conflicts, and other global strife, the #mood we breathe is one of distress. Cvetkovich (2012) proposed a perspective of depression as a collective "anxiety and numbness" best understood on the societal level. Although I hesitate to embrace depression as an entirely social phenomenon, I find value in Cvetkovich's diagnosis of the social dimensions of depression and note that her analysis resonates with Thomas Rickert's call to attend to the ambient nature of rhetoric, even while it relates to the way depression is handled in meme renderings. For Rickert (2013), rhetoric is "the complex entwinement of discourse, mood, things, and environment" (p. 31), and as internet-era rhetoric, depression memes illustrate contemporary life's undercurrent of anguish through their pervasive usage of depression symptoms as stand-ins for generalized suffering (and vice versa). More particularly, these lenses serve as useful ways to understand the internet's usage of "big sad" and "mood" from a scholarly perspective; where internet users are describing the phenomenon thusly, scholars have begun to do the same.

Memes are joking commonplaces; as internet-era rhetoric, they are instantly recognizable as trending, repeated, and shareable social media posts. Although Dawkins' (1976) perspective of memes refers to all cultural tropes (including phrases, images, ideas, beliefs, dance moves, and anything else that replicates in a social body), I focus on the specific phenomenon known as the "internet meme," which designates a combination of image and text shared and re-shared in a digital space (Dynel, 2016; Hahner, 2013; Huntington, 2016). In designating "internet memes" I refer to any digital image that is re-purposed and shared. Although memes often take the form of video, audio, slang, jargon, or other repeatable content, I focus on the vast array of image+text memes that circulate through digital spaces. This format is most often referred to as a "meme," designated by the countless social media pages dedicated to creating, sharing, and re-sharing.

For the purposes of my study, then, memes refer to any oft-repeated, recognizable internet image, usually with text added. Interestingly, the Urban Dictionary's top definition for "memes" is "The cure of depression" (Urban Dictionary, 2019). The second definition reads: "Memes are graceful, exquisite entities bestowed upon us, filthy peasants, which are sporadically known to drift one into a sea of existential crises. This is also an exemplary method of eliminating depression once and for all" (Urban Dictionary, 2019). Urban Dictionary definitions are curated by user votes; of the top five user-generated definitions for memes, four of them include a reference to depression or suicide. The important linkage between depression and memes is already established by internet users; I now seek to understand them as rhetorical phenomena.

Typically (though not always), memes are jokes. A standard meme is a short, quippy blurb (often incorporating both image and text) that satirizes a social phenomenon (Dynel, 2016; Hahner, 2013; Huntington, 2016). Memes vary widely in their sophistication, nuance, and niche, and require a certain level of outside knowledge to understand the reference. When I refer to "memes," I mean this type of digitally circulated image that is instantly recognizable as a meme by internet users. Although other memetic texts (such as beliefs, ideas, jargon, etc.) are certainly memes, I focus on internet memes for their popularity in contemporary digital spheres, their meaningful usage of depression as a trope, and for the practicality of research purposes. Memes' joking format allows users to critique, analyze, express, indicate, or otherwise address salient topics quickly and with emphasis. Viewing memes as "expressions can tell scholars much about what makes sense to different publics and which energies, tendencies, desires, and affections speak to the perceived social field, and thereby move people, tickling their funny bones and encapsulating their anxieties" (Jenkins, 2016, p. 463). That is, memes utilize older versions of themselves to make playful judgements about their subject matter, and yet the effects of humor are not strictly *persuasive*. In a meta-analysis on humor and persuasion, Walter et al. (2018) explored the effects of relatability and its impact on knowledge, attitudes, and behavior. Interestingly, humor was found to be less efficacious on persuasion than on knowledge; that is, humor teaches.

Indeed, “ambiguous humor often impedes persuasion, as it leaves much more room for selective perception and individual interpretation” (Walter et al., 2018, p. 363).

Memes, then, can be considered playful judgements of cultural tropes, and they can educate viewers on how the world “works” from a particular perspective. Jenkins' (2016) usage of “anxieties” is especially important; although memes are certainly humorous, they can also express serious political, social, or personal meanings. Significantly, “memes visualise the experience and encumbering nature of depressive symptoms, which for many may be difficult to verbalise. Therefore, by sharing and observing depressive memes, depressed individuals may theoretically form social and emotional bonds” (Akram et al., 2020, p. 8). These examples illustrate how memes as expressions can illuminate meanings in social contexts, with an emphasis on their ability to connect users through mental/emotional worldviews.

Depression memes purportedly utilize depression as the butt of the joke, and yet draw upon vast discourses of knowledges about what it means to be sane, insane, healthy, and unhealthy. Figure 1.2, significantly, never mentions depression by name, nor does it refer to specific symptoms, instead referring vaguely to “feelings” and “mood.” When I show this picture to students and colleagues, the response is almost always a pause followed by a short laugh with a wry comment of bitter agreement. Figure 1.2 is a meta-meme: as a meme about memes, it depicts a relatable experience through a relatable format. More particularly, however, it illustrates a meta-discourse about depression online (and, increasingly, offline), that emphasizes the social aspects—perhaps to the detriment of individual experience.

Students, in particular, discourse at length about how mental illness is glamorized online; memes are only one way to do so. The example in Figure 1.2 also describes the ineffability of the experience of depression and the ability of memes to better express one's symptoms. Importantly, it refers to the habitual expression of symptomatic emotions through interacting with meme posts online. The meme depicts several dimensions of struggle: the inability to express emotion, the implied assumption that negative emotions are on the table, the difficulty of understanding one's own emotions, to start. It also requires knowledge of therapy, a familiarity with the "meme pictures" referred to, and a recognition of the same ineffability of experience in order to fully relate to the joke.

These memetic tropes, according to memes and colloquial chat, online and off, illustrate the popular circulatory trend of visual humor normalizing depression symptoms (for better or for worse). Indeed, the digital realms are full of a "never-ending barrage of little micro-jokes," of which we have become serious connoisseurs (Jennings, 2018, p. 21). The "energies" of internet memes are useful rhetorical objects of study, as jokes hold significance in our current global moment. In a popular work on the rise of comedy in American culture, gameshow celebrity and comedian Ken Jennings explored contemporary culture's emphasis on humor, such that it permeates all aspects of social life, from the mundane to the serious. Similarly, humor is permeating the way online users discuss depression symptoms, both on the individual and societal levels (as examples throughout will demonstrate).

Figure 1.2

"Mood"

Therapist: and how does that make you feel?

"I am not very good at describing my emotions, maybe you could just hold up a bunch of meme pictures until I see one that I would normally comment the word "mood" on?"

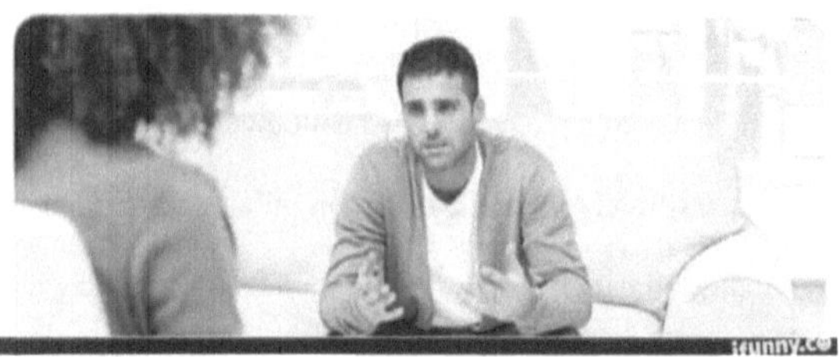

From a scholarly perspective, Wickberg (1998) traced humor's rise in importance from the early days of settlement and democracy until the present era; he noted that while a sense of humor in a political candidate seemed trite and irrelevant in times past, political candidates now must have a sense of humor to be taken seriously. Flowers and Young (2010) noted the importance of satire in political campaigns as they explored the "confluence of visual and verbal dimensions of political communication and contextual elements" in *Saturday Night Live* (*SNL*) parodies of political candidates (p. 49). Through the circulation of parodies on the internet, *SNL* jokes had a real impact on the 2008 election when they shifted viewers' voting perspectives (Flowers & Young, 2010).

Humorous images have historically served as satirical expressions. For instance, Alston and Platt (1969), analyzed religious cartoons from 1930 to 1968 and found that comedic images make judgements by "criticizing or ridiculing deviant behavior" (p. 218). More recently, internet jokes stand as playful and disruptive strategies to subvert traditional engagement through artful participation in existing trends (Harold, 2004). By contrasting a modern playful rhetoric with the traditional, logical and industrial rhetoric of former times, Harold elucidates a particular kind of persuasion built upon chaotic critique. Harold utilizes three case studies of online collectives who organize for the purpose of radical activism through pranking. That is, "pranking repatterns commercial rhetoric . . . by strategically augmenting and utilizing the precious resources the contemporary media ecology affords" (Harold, 2004, p. 208).

As humorous disruptions spread across a culture, they invoke new kinds of meaning through the upending of older rhetorical modes. In Harold's (2004) examples, pranks "reconfigure the very structures of meaning and production on which corporate media and advertising depend" (p. 209). Through the alteration of existing images, Harold's case studies illustrate a tension between seemingly chaotic images and their rhetorical power. Pertinently, Walter et al. (2018) found that "humorous appeals are best suited for educated, younger audiences" (p. 362), a crucial population for the study of depression memes. Further, Walter et al. emphasized a need to study humor on social media due to "affordances such as interactivity and the endorsement of messages by friends" (p. 364). Indeed, "given the centrality of humor to discourse on social media, it is imperative to examine the effects of humorous messages when they are packaged into new media formats" (Walter et al., 2018, p. 364).

Sarcasm, in particular, serves as a powerful tool for memetic humor. According to Harvey et al. (2019), both pro- and anti-vaccine memes utilized an appeal to rationality by instructing their viewers on how to view the opposite position. That is, "sarcastic humor provides a more socially acceptable way over direct criticism to elaborate on the negative stereotypes of the out-group and to enhance in-group cohesion by justifying in-group superiority" (Harvey et al., 2019, p. 1020). Sarcasm in depression memes provokes an interesting dichotomy; by identifying an out-group (that is, non-depressed people), depression memes might designate an in-group. That is, perhaps depression memes provide a sense of belonging in online groups. At any rate, "people may use sarcasm to protect their reputation while indirectly criticizing others," (Harvey et al., 2019, p. 1020), a fascinating consideration for depression memes.

Additionally, depression memes' popularity exists in an economy of virality. In our contemporary sphere, motion eclipses content, as we attribute "viral" objects value for their sheer popularity. Van Horn, Beveridge, and Morey (2016) traced Twitter content to determine "whether content merits trending in the first place seems to now be secondary to the question of whether content has gained attention" (par. 9). They developed a "virality threshold" to explore the extent to which certain trends "stick," or whether they are mere flashes in the pan of popular attention—including journalistic and news media attention. They note that "the hyper-circulatory nature of viral information should reflect the underlying social attention itself, which in turn can lead to reiteration and recirculation" (Van Horn, Beveridge, & Morey, 2016, par. 44). That is, information in this historical moment is valued for the mere premise of being shared, rather than for any inherent worth. Depression memes carry their own importance through their popularity.

Sarcasm, virality, and other complicating factors in the value of memes as cultural objects points to an additional factor: ambivalence. Phillips and Milner (2017) traced the significance of what they term "the ambivalent internet" across a variety of platforms and examples, arguing, on the whole, that internet texts are:

> simultaneously antagonistic and social, creative and disruptive, humorous and barbed, the satirization of products, antagonization of celebrities, and creation of questionable fan art, along with countless other examples that permeate contemporary online participation, are too unwieldy, too variable across specific cases, to be essentialized as this as opposed to that. (p. 10).

Phillips and Milner use "ambivalence" to describe a particular kind of blended polyvocality and polyvalence, mixed with multiplicities of meaning and a great deal of variability in online spaces. Indeed, Poe's Law, as defined by Phillips and Milner (2017), is "an online axiom stipulating the difficulty of distinguishing irony from earnestness in public conversation online" (p. 51).

Ambivalence, overall, refers to the internet's polymorphic treatment of feelings. Mixed feelings are communicated online through posts, discourses, interactions, and other rhetorical texts. These messages suggest meanings and feelings that can be interpreted as good, bad, and indifferent, as well as pointless, meaningful, playful, and serious. Ambivalence is a kind of exaggerated ambiguity, and the internet is an abundant breeding ground for these kinds of ambivalent readings. Ambivalence is a key concept for a study of depression memes because memes are notoriously hard to "pin down"; memes use double entendre, ironies, sarcasm, etc., as humorous devices, which makes memes' meanings ambiguous, especially among different viewers. An ambivalent view of the internet takes the possibility of ambiguous meanings into account, suggesting that memes contain symbolic elements that defy a single or dominant interpretation.

That is, although the interpretations of depression memes are highly ambivalent, there will be some limitations between those in the depression memes community and those without. As illustrated by Akram et al. (2020), depression memes are perceived as more relatable, humorous, and impactful by those who actually possess depression symptoms, as opposed to those who do not. Although ambivalence allows for nearly infinite interpretations of rhetorical texts (Phillips & Milner, 2017), depression memes provide a particularly interesting example because they are interpreted in layers of recognition by those more familiar with the symptoms of depression "IRL" and the rhetoric of depression in memes online.

Further, they provide a uniquely ambivalent interpretation of the world by juxtaposing humor and suffering – upon which the joke usually hinges. Depression memes are both filled with "mixed" feelings (elements that are simultaneously humorous and serious) and juxtapose the humorous and the serious. Throughout this book, I will explain how depression memes' ambivalence reflects contain a constrained, rather than entirely open, polysemy: they offer humorous opportunities to connect with others who experience depression while inviting those who do not suffer from depression to understand the affective experience of the illness. The latter individuals, understandably, may not find the memes quite as humorous as those who experience depression—an assumption empirically verified by Akram et al. (2020)—but the memes' unstated connections to circulating popular discourses allows each group of viewers to "get," albeit with different interpretations, the memes' humor. Those who suffer from depression can find perceived social support, a lightening of mood, and a means of regulating their emotions in the memes' stark humor (Akram, et al., 2020), while those who do not suffer from depression can more vividly feel the suffering of those who do—even if they might be shocked by their perceptions of the memes' humor.

A pre-internet meme that cannot be traced to any one author (although it is attributed variously to Mark Twain, E.B. White, André Maurois, and Marty Feldman) compares explaining a joke to dissecting a frog. The analogy has been made different times in different ways, but the gist is that if you explain a joke or dissect a frog, you gain knowledge but kill the joke and the frog. Many memes have been "killed" in the process of this book, but in the dissecting of them I have teased out ambiguities in the memes and the circulations they inhabit/perpetuate. Just as the quip about jokes and frogs cannot be traced to any original source, memes are what I term "deep" rhetoric: the origins are too deeply rooted to trace. Memes, after all, have lives of their own. Throughout this book, I dissect a number of memes, but their ambivalence ensures that my dissection can never approach a thorough reading. Still, memes' complexity makes a partial dissection worthwhile as part of an ongoing scholarly attempt to define memes as rhetorical objects.

Ambient Memes, Ambient Depression

Although internet memes are relatively new, memes in general are old. Meme studies often reference Dawkins' (1976) original perspective of "the selfish gene," later concretized by Blackmore (1999), who viewed a meme as a replicator "drifting clumsily about in its primeval soup of culture" (p. 5). Viewed through the memetic perspective, memes are random, viral replicators of cultural information through a biological metaphor of evolution. Indeed, from the original memetic perspective, "just as genes propagate themselves in the gene pool . . . so memes propagate themselves in the memepool by leaping from brain to brain via a process which, in the broad sense, can be called imitation" (Dawkins, 1976, p. 192). Popular definitions are similar, as the sub-Reddit on memes defines them thusly: "Memes! A way of describing cultural information being shared. An element of a culture or system of behavior that may be considered to be passed from one individual to another by nongenetic means, especially imitation" (r/memes, 2020).

From the Dawkins (1976) perspective, memes are viral, random, mindless copies of previous information, each taking on a mind and will of its own and with very little, if any, human agency in the mix. However, more recent meme scholars explore the argumentative properties of internet memes and their rhetorical power to re-purpose old content and create something uniquely new (Hahner, 2013; Huntington, 2016). That is, Dawkins' (1976) original memetic perspective fails to grasp the important nuances of internet memes as rhetorical objects. Memes, as primarily visual forms of rhetoric, can be understood as depictors of abstract concepts; knowledges, beliefs, concepts, cultural tropes, and other taken-for-granted social phenomena are embedded in memes in specific ways.

From a rhetorical standpoint, memes are "neatly packaged visual arguments" (Huntington, 2016, p. 91) and viewing them as such allows a more fruitful explication than viewing them as purely memetic. For instance, Cannizzaro (2016) favors a semiotic view of memes by viewing them as relational instead of discrete, translation instead of transmission, and habit instead of virality. Similarly, Grundlingh (2018) views memes as speech acts, demonstrating that memes accomplish particular functions beyond mere "jokes," such as critiquing a political figure or presenting serious opinions. Indeed, scholars are not quite satisfied with the Dawkins (1976) perspective; it does not quite fit.

Although memes might seem random to non-memers, practiced memers are intimately familiar with the codes, combinations, and structures of various meme styles. Katz and Shifman (2017), in a study of "nonsense as a generative force of affective meaning," discussed "nonsense" as playful subversiveness—not merely the aimless replication proposed by the Dawkins tradition (p. 839). For Katz and Shifman (2017), "memetic nonsense . . . creates a system with a set of rules which govern expression" (p. 839). Thus, instead of thinking of memes as random, viral replicators, memes are intricate renderings of specific rhetorical codes. Understanding memes as primarily visual rhetoric allows a more meaningful appreciation of their content, as a rhetorical perspective provides a lens to view memes as in relation with other memes and other communicative structures. Memes, of course, rely on verbal elements, which I explore more in Chapter Two; for now, though, memes' visual components invite closer consideration into the persuasive abilities of visual rhetorical texts, particularly as a way of understanding memes.

In particular, depression memes provide visual adaptations of offline suffering represented in online spaces. The ambivalent participation in memeing about depression symptoms in online spaces illuminates a particular kind of discourse around mental health (or the lack thereof) through playful schema of memetic tropes. Mixed feelings, as portrayed online, participate in a complex, multi-layered discourse surrounding wellness and illness in contemporary society.

Memes, thus, can serve as indicators of both an individual's experience of depression and an international #mood of suffering, best understood through an ambient perspective. Ambience, as defined by Rickert (2013), uses atmosphere as a metaphor to describe rhetoric as the very rhetorical "air" we breathe. In other words, ambience is a question of "wakefulness" (via Heidegger) or perception or recognition of environment, rather than any one entity within that environment (Rickert, 2013, p. 4). Ambience views rhetoric as "revealing and doing—doing as revealing and revealing as doing—and hence integral to our dwelling in the world" (Rickert, 2013, p. 33). Memes are particularly good candidates for an ambient reading of the world; their ability to succinctly-yet-complexly summarize an issue makes them ripe for an ambient ambivalent analysis, particularly through memes' uncanny ability to permeate online and offline worlds. To appreciate memes' contribution to our ambient rhetorical environment, we also need to recognize how a collective mood of suffering circulates between and through both online and offline spaces.

As depression memes replicate online, depression symptoms grow offline. Statistically speaking, humans are being diagnosed in exponential numbers, particularly among the teen and twenty-something population that typically uses memes, and suicide is also increasing in that age group (Curtin & Heron, 2019; Hedegaard, Curtin, & Warner, 2020). A recent Pew poll demonstrated that 70% of teens in the United States believe anxiety and depression to be a "major concern" (Horowitz & Graf, 2019). A longitudinal study of American university students found a steady up-ward trend in depressive symptoms between 1938 and 2007 (Twenge et al., 2010), and my proposed data collection period coincided with a global pandemic that increased a tensioned online dialogue of stress, worry, and overwhelm. In short, individual and collective suffering is a significant topic in online spaces and is facilitated through conversations about depression through memes.

Simultaneously, lay sources note the trend of social media as a glamorizer of mental health disorders. In merely one example, Premack (2016), in an article for *The Ringer* online, discussed the "shared sadness" found on Tumblr that glamorizes a particular aesthetic of melancholy. Scholarly sources have argued this as well: in a content analysis of 20 popular Imgur posts, Hale (2019) explored the ways that commenters provided social support to users who posted about their depression, connecting through shared symptoms. Similarly, Jadayel, Medlej, and Jadayel (2017) found that through the ministrations of social media, "many teenagers and young adults now see mental disorders as relatable, normal and desirable, while people actually diagnosed with any mental health disorder might get a false impression that what they are experiencing is normal and common" (pp. 474-475). Interestingly, Hale (2019) suggested that "depression-related discourse within Imgur is simultaneously supportive and humorous" (p. 9), emphasizing the social support present in the comments of images on the platform.

In particular, scholars have explored mental health in terms of adolescents and emergent adults, as these populations are particularly at risk for mental illness and spend the most time online (Miguel et al., 2017; Windler et al., 2019). In a study of youth aged 14 to 26, Windler et al. (2019) found that moderators in mental health support groups were able to promote healthy attitudes and perceptions of mental health online. However, the vast majority of the web remains unmoderated, and promotion of disordered behaviors online continues.

On the one hand, social media posts about mental health might disseminate important information and reduce stigma, if practitioners are mindful of their presentation (Yap et al., 2017). On the other hand, social media discourse can further stigmatize sufferers and present misinformation to the general public. This ambivalence is illustrated in Pan et al.'s (2018) three-year study of social media posts on *Sina Weibo*. Pan et al. discussed the power of social media as a shaper of public opinion around mental health disorders. Popular beliefs about depression, they noted, frame sufferers as weak and dramatic and in need of help. In particular, "stories of ordinary users, especially those with depression and those with first-hand experience with depression, may have impact on opinion leaders, organizations, and mass media" (Pan et al., 2018, p. 9). These findings demonstrate that online discussions of mental health have a powerful impact on public perceptions.

Further, some posts glamorize mental illness through the promotion of self-harm, suicide, or other dangerous behaviors, and content analyses have demonstrated that social media platforms are spaces whereon users fail to discourage and even promote injurious mental health behavior. For instance, Miguel et al. (2017) noted that only one in 10 and one in 20 posts actively discouraged self-harm; the rest were "saturated with graphic content and negative self-evaluations, lacking in content discouraging deliberate self-injury, and rarely providing recovery resources" (p. 789). In another example, Eliseo-Arras, Brous, and Sheppard (2019) explored "the wide variety of people experiencing emotional distress that are turning to Tumblr for various reasons," which, they suggested, "is creating an abundance of categories that are either negative in nature or related to mental illness, but very few positive or helping categories" (p. 208). Thus, social media platforms create negative portrayals of mental health through discourse and might do more harm than good when it comes to describing and interpreting what it means to suffer from a mental illness—even as they also potentially help those who suffer from depression.

Corresponding discourses provide an important point of comparison. Importantly, images are important and widespread components of social media posts (Carrotte, Prichard, & Lim, 2017; Wick & Harriger, 2017) and mental illness is often portrayed online through visual means (Miguel et al., 2017; Eliseo-Arras et al., 2019). A similar example can be found in fitness posts online; as social media chatter about exercise, weight, body image, and physical attractiveness portrays particular ways of being through photographic representation (Boepple et al., 2017; Deighton-Smith & Bell, 2018; Lydecker et al., 2016; Tiggeman & Zacardo, 2018; Webb et al., 2017). Fitness posts (often called "fitspiration") provide images of idealized body types as inspiration to social media followers who might choose to attain a similar body shape through working out or dieting. Similarly, pro-eating disorder (pro-ED) posts portray eating disorders as "normal" and healthy lifestyles to be achieved through dieting and exercise, an extreme form of social support in online spaces (Cavazos-Rehg et al., 2019; Pila et al., 2016; Simpson & Mazzeo, 2016; Talbot et al., 2017). In posts about fitness and thinness, images are used as markers of glamorized, normalized extremity; that is, the very thin and the very muscular are portrayed as desirable and healthy, whether they are attainable and realistic or not.

Fitspiration posts and pro-ED posts provide a parallel example to depression memes because they are another source of the normalized and idealized self as portrayed in online spaces, which has a complex relationship to what it means to suffer in the digital age. In particular, Deighton-Smith and Bell (2018) found that fitspiration "promotes unrealistic body ideals beyond those that are achievable for most" social media viewers, which might be harmful to self-image (p. 479). Similarly, Simpson and Mazzeo (2016), in a study of fitspiration posts in conjunction with social cognitive theory, argued that the "visible display of engagement furthers the acceptance of unrealistic body image ideals and adoption of the idealized behaviors" found on social media posts (p. 565). That is, images of extremely thin and muscular bodies online encourage viewers to engage in fitness behaviors that achieve a certain ideal, which is dictated by the "normal" bodies portrayed on social media platforms. They offer space for ambivalent interpretations, though, because those who do not subscribe to the posts' realities can see the glamorization of unhealthy behaviors.

Importantly, the examples listed in this section participate in an ambivalent discussion about what "healthy" means. Like Ahmed's (2010) suggestion about the imposed necessity of happiness in post-modernity, visual rhetoric online provides a plethora of information about what it means to be "normal" in a complex, multi-faceted series of discourses around wellness and unwellness, health and illness. As social media discourse holds a significant influence over public perceptions, "mental health professionals must recognize the rapidly changing landscape of adolescent media consumption, influences, and social interaction as they may pertain to self-harm patterns" (Miguel et al., 2017, p. 789). Scholars, too, could do more to understand the interaction of users and mental health, which is an intricate and intertwined relationship. Indeed, studies report that "social media can serve as both a positive element of harm-reduction and social support and a negative function of perpetrating self-harm and shame" (Eliseo-Arras et al., 2019, p. 208). More research is needed to tease out the complex roles of social media discourse and mental illness, especially through visual representations.

Thus far, I have painted a portrait of depression memes as rhetorical objects embedded in an ambivalent discourse not easily dis-entangled from other discourses, practices, and rhetorics online and offline. As such, depression memes cannot, and should not, be separated from an understanding of suffering that is experienced in offline spaces; as Rickert (2013) emphasized in his discussions of attunement and ambience, our rhetorical environment takes in and breathes out rhetorical discourses from both spaces. Even more importantly, the examples in this section also rely on situated understandings of the world, what Rickert (2013) would call attunement to globalized discourses. Depression—as experienced, shared, and constructed through social and rhetorical means—is not solely an internal or mental phenomenon (Cvetkovich, 2012). In a time of complex, globalized discourse surrounding wellness and unwellness, theoretical work on memeing must take into account multiple, complex factors of rhetoricity (as I have described throughout). I ask three research questions that seek to understand what depression memes "reveal and do" (Rickert, 2013) in our contemporary rhetorical environment:

> RQ1: What are the affective dimensions of depression memes?
>
> RQ2: What topics do depression memes circulate?
>
> RQ3: What do depression memes communicate about contemporary cultural conditions?

By discussing one research question per chapter, I build upon each concept as part of my ultimate goal of making a case for memes as the ambient "scaffolding" (Rickert, 2013) of our current understandings of depression. I seek to understand how depression memes both "reveal and do" (Rickert, 2013) discursive meanings of sane and insane, healthy and ill, well and unwell.

In Chapter 2, I describe my theoretical commitments to Rickert's (2013) theory of ambient rhetoric, which he defined as "attunement that can generate various kinds of knowledge, in particular a knowledge of how the world gives back, as it were, or how the world transcendent of human thought and power is integral to how life takes shape" (Rickert, 2013, p. 27). Utilizing ambience as a framework allows a broad view of memes as particles in our rhetorical environment; rather than isolated, random packages of nonsense, they are intricate, complex pieces of a globalized network of discourse. Rickert draws upon literature from affect and circulation studies, which are relevant to meme research in their own right: I first outline circulation studies as a pivotal lens to understand memes and then trace circulation through affect studies. Then, I draw upon Rickert's ambient rhetoric as a fit construct for meme studies and set forth his usage of both circulation and affect as theoretical support for ambience. I emphasize Rickert's use of Heidegger's *Stimmung*, new materialism, and the Cartesian split as crucial elements to the discourse of depression online.

In Chapter 3, I explore the representation of affect through depression memes' enthymematic claims about depression as an experiential state of being, in response to RQ1, which asks about the affective dimensions of depression memes. Memes represent important cultural assumptions surrounding mental health in contemporary digital culture as expressed through humorous critique online. As visual arguments, memes show viewers what mental illness "looks" like, and their implicit premises require the viewer to fill in the gaps between the verbal and nonverbal elements of the meme. In short, I describe what depression memes "reveal" (Rickert, 2013) about our contemporary understandings of depression, as a baseline for my subsequent arguments about embeddedness and ambience.

In Chapter 4, I explore depression as a *topos* circulated through memes online in response to RQ2, which interrogates depression as a topic as portrayed through memes. Memes are circular, participatory globules of discourse, and as such provide a unique window into current social "moods" as depicted by depression memes online. Scholars have linked the enthymeme with the *topos* (for instance, see Dyck, 2002), and viewing memes as enthymematic *topoi* provides a nuanced explication of memes, which operate based on commonplace assumptions and implicit meanings. Combining *topos* with enthymeme allows us to unpack the cultural discourses that we rely upon to make sense of them. Memes as enthymematic *topoi* "do" (Rickert, 2013) significant discourses about depression and suffering in our contemporary moment. In this chapter, I argue that the *topos* of depression online is that of *embeddedness*—since discourses and cultures of depression are circulating so intimately, they are fully integrated with the online sphere's daily communication (rather than a fringe or edge discourse).

In Chapter 5, I analyze memes as attunement to suffering in our contemporary moment in response to RQ3, which asks about depression memes as carriers of discourse. In other words, how do our views of suffering (as expressed through depression memes) represent the zeitgeist or *Stimmung* of the 21st century? With Cvetkovich (2012), I "explore…depression as a cultural discourse and the pervasive and widespread contemporary representation of it as a medical disease that can be treated pharmacologically" (p. 13). Pushing back against that cultural discourse, Cvetkovich understands depression as a "public feeling," one which represents a blockage of rhetorical movement. Similarly, I suggest that depression memes circulate an ambient, affective reality of normalized, collective suffering, even while they attempt to release the cultural blockages they describe. The result is an ambivalent, deep-structure understanding of depression that both loosens and tightens the hyper-medicalized understanding of depression that pervades the Western world today.

Finally, in the concluding chapter, I suggest that memes are furnishings for our contemporary "dwelling" (Rickert, 2013) in depression; we shape and mold them as they simultaneously shape and mold us. A more critical literacy of digital rhetoric is merely one path; systemic changes, it seems, are necessary. By utilizing digital rhetoric as a tool for understanding what it means to be a post-modern citizen, we can begin to shape ambient landscapes (or memescapes) for future generations.

Chapter 2: Ambient Memeing

In an analysis of social media usage in the Cairo revolution, Edwards (2011) explicated the uneasy balance between *hisa* (chaos, noise, movement) and *zhama* (blockage) as expressed through circulations of protest on social media. For revolutionaries, the frustration of government blockades, or *zhama*, could be circumnavigated by social media communications, or *hisa*, which allowed freedom of expression and organization in a context that sought to prevent movement during curfews and lockdowns (Edwards, 2011). I propose that depression, as a public feeling, erects blockages to social and political health that depression memes seek to circumnavigate through circulations of affective experience. Meanwhile, depression memes explore the blockage and release of depression as affective suffering through memetic expression.

In rhetorical studies, scholars trace a line between reading for meaning or motion, and most accomplish only one or the other (Edwards, 2011). Meaning, in a rhetorical context, focuses on the situated claims made by a given text, while motion traces a text's movement through discursive realms (Edwards, 2011). In Edwards' (2011) view, a tension exists between the circulation of texts and their individual expressions, as each focus results in different kinds of rhetorical meaning-making; he asks, how can we read for both motion *and* meaning? I echo Edwards' question and provide one potential answer: memes as moving targets in a swirling mass of online discourse, and their individual meanings hold impact for their creators, viewers, and sharers. That is, the experience of viewing a meme (a fleeting, inert, visual expression) is contained within a vast, complex universe of motion (chaotic, tensioned, and complex). In other words, memes encapsulate both meaning and motion through their eloquent combinations of movement and *in situ* claims.

To read depression memes as both meaning and motion, I propose to utilize two rhetorical lenses: ambience and enthymeme. While ambience provides a lens to view memes as part of circulatory relationships (i.e., in motion), they first require a meaningful critique of their situated meanings. As noted in the previous chapter, the *in situ* claims of memes have been understood through a variety of rhetorical perspectives. For the purpose of this work, I propose the enthymeme as a more effective appreciation of the subtly nuanced layers of meaning contained therein, especially when we consider the how visual properties of enthymeme open up possibilities for interpretations of the words they contain.

Memes as Enthymemes

Visual rhetoric provides an alternative to Dawkins' (1976) memetic perspective. Gallagher and Zagacki (2007), in an exploration of Civil Rights activism photos in *Life* magazine, explored how images make abstract concepts knowable, specifically how "photographs brought what had been previously invisible, in light of the abstract, de-personalized nature of the rhetoric, into clear focus" (p. 125). Similarly, Bacon (2007) noted the power of African American newspaper writers to frame blackness and whiteness in the anti-colonization debate through photographs more clearly than through verbal means. In Gallagher and Zagacki's and Bacon's examples, the difficulty of expressing racial tension was in some ways answered by visuality. As depression memes move through digital spaces, they satirize taken-for-granted beliefs by calling them to our attention in impactful, visual ways. The worn-out adage that "a picture is worth a thousand words" is eclipsed by the notion that memes use pictures *and* words – and they are arranged in meaningful ways that make what is ineffable, effable.

Pertinently, images represent constitutive rhetoric in circulation. For instance, Gallagher and Zagacki (2007) described photos as "depictions of social experience that are recognizable to common audiences and that add moral import to the decisions or developments before them" (p. 127). That is, images make concrete the abstract and make knowable the unknowable through their circulation through social groups. By drawing attention to "deep rules" in a societal body, visual rhetoric can draw out unspoken concepts and make them understandable in ways not readily expressed (Gallagher & Zagacki, 2007). Similarly, the "deep rules" of certain social spheres play out in internet memes, as users circulate them through discursive realms.

Although scholars have viewed memes from other rhetorical lenses, such as semiotics (for instance, see Cannizzaro, 2016 or Grundlingh, 2018), I propose an additional alternative in partnership with visual rhetoric. For contemporary scholars, Aristotle's enthymeme is "an argument that has one or more premises . . . not explicitly stated in the text" (Walton, 2001, p. 93). I propose a theory of memes as visual enthymeme, which will better encapsulate how memes function as units of culture through a reliance on implicit knowledge of outside experiences.

Generally, utilizing enthymeme as a construct allows us to grasp the implicative intricacies of memes, which hide the "deep rules" of society between the visual and the verbal. Although a few lay sources (for instance, see Chandler, 2015) and one scholarly source (Collins, 2015) link the enthymeme with internet memes (Chen, 2018: Kennerly & Pfister, 2018), most see the connection as negligible (Kennerly & Pfister, 2018). Indeed, Kennerly and Pfister (2018) discuss the enthymeme as a homonym to the term "meme" but emphasize its different classical language roots as a side note in their scholarly project to "humble" the "selfish gene" (p. 209). Although the connection may be etymologically negligible, the rhetorical functions of enthymeme and internet memes are identical, as I demonstrate below.

To my knowledge, only one scholarly article uses enthymeme as an analytical construct for the internet meme (see Collins, 2015). Collins (2015) analyzed sexist memes as dangerous expressions of gender norms, using the enthymeme as a construct to unpack bigoted humor in online spaces. For Collins, internet memes are "perilous" because they require sexist behavior to get the joke; the memes perpetuate sexism because their missing premises insist upon certain knowledges. Collins further argued that counter-memes are a possible combat for sexism in online spaces, as enthymematic understanding of memes can allow for re-purposing sexist memes for more pro-social intents through enthymematic persuasion. Following Collins' example, I seek to unpack the in-between persuasive assumptions of depression memes, which require their viewers to grasp extensive cultural knowledges to appreciate the joke. These cultural knowledges point to discursive understandings of contemporary suffering as presented online.

Traditional rhetorical scholarship has understood the enthymeme as a truncated syllogism that operates based on logical proof (Cronkhite, 1966). That perspective has been critiqued by a number of scholars, however, on a variety of fronts. Some scholars argue that Aristotle's original conception of the enthymeme has been lost to the Western understanding of rhetoric and must be re-envisioned in order to better encapsulate the power of the enthymeme in contemporary rhetoric (Cronkhite, 1966). Specifically, scholars have worked to push back against the traditional assumption that an enthymeme is merely a "truncated syllogism," but instead an implicit argument made by creating common understanding with the audience (Aune, 2003); in other words, the audience is invited to make certain assumptions to fill in the gaps. In particular, enthymemes are "used to encapsulate arguments" (Aune, 2003, p. 306) rather than spell them out through lengthy logical proofs.

Traditionally, rhetorical scholars have understood Aristotle's enthymeme as a "deductive rhetorical argument" (Cronkhite, 1966, p. 134) that relies on reading between the lines of explicit premises. Hidden within the explicit premises are implicit premises, sometimes understood by scholars as deliberately omitted premises. Understanding the implicit premises between explicit premises has allowed scholars to illuminate persuasive texts as innately convincing, almost without the audience's agentic consent. That is, an enthymematic argument is one that influences its viewer at the subconscious level, before any logical reasoning has even been attempted.

Enthymeme comes from the Greek terms *En* and *Thymos,* which together designate an assumption made "in [the] mind" (Miller & Bee, 1972, p. 202; Walton, 2001). As such, enthymemes can represent a way of knowing. Prenosil (2012) argued for an ontological theory of enthymemes, noting that "the enthymeme's deep grammar is one of relationality among entities" (p. 280). This relationality, Prenosil (2012) argued, creates a complex and multi-layered relationship that can make powerful claims. According to Prenosil (2012), "the enthymeme is not a series of language propositions of analytical philosophy, but rather an endless hybrid reality that eludes our definition. The 'missing premises' of the enthymeme become a vast, 'dark reservoir' of possibilities for rhetorical encounters" (p. 298). Prenosil (2012) argued, then, that the premises are not "missing" but rather "hiding" within that network of possibilities. Similarly, internet memes exist in a complex relationship to other forms of rhetoric, their viewers, and to each other.

Thus, the internet meme as enthymeme illuminates memes' function as shared and implicit knowledge that circulates through a network. Scott (2002) explored the ways that the "enthymeme not only plays on an audience's assumptions but can also help shape those assumptions" (p. 61). In the case of mental health memes, audience members must already have some preconceived notions about memes, mental health, and the meme's specific context in order to recognize, grasp, and agree with the argument (although the entire process takes place in milliseconds of cognitive processing). In turn, these arguments build on the viewer's preconceived notions and experiences of mental health and become part of that viewer's understanding of what mental health means in contemporary culture. As a result, depression memes possess ambivalence; depending upon the types of enthymematic connections drawn, viewers of these memes may interpret them as "speaking truth" to fellow sufferers or trivializing a serious condition.

Rhetorical work on enthymeme has typically stated the explicit premises of a rhetorical work and then analytically un-packed the implicit premises from in-between (for example, see Scott, 2002). Through an explication of memes and counter-memes, Collins (2015) demonstrated the ability of memes to enthymematically influence belief and behavior. Van Horn, Beveridge, and Morey (2016) noted that in an attention economy where viral trends abound, "the question of whether content merits trending in the first place seems to now be secondary to the question of whether content has gained attention" (par. 9). In general, internet memes already have implicit premises due to and resulting from their virality before we even begin to analyze their explicit premises:

1. This meme is viral
2. Viral memes have value
3. Therefore, this meme is valuable

Naturally, the relative value of a given meme will depend on its popularity. By definition, however, any given meme has been shared at least once, giving it implicit value through its status as an object worth sharing. The mental health memes in my sample, thus, hold value, and therefore they hold power.

Some scholars have begun to study how circulatory enthymemes make powerful arguments via their movement through a social body. For instance, Cos and Martin (2013) noted that meaning is contextually based—that is, "not found in words themselves but from the collected and remembered experiences we have" (p. 1700). Cos and Martin used the example of Obama's empty chair circulated through online spaces with a wide variety of interpretations, depending on the political affiliation of the viewer. In their example, images of the empty chair took on polysemic meanings, depending on the viewer's political leanings, background, and experience with the meme. The emptiness of the chair was significant, as it required a mental "filling in" of the chair in order to grasp its meaning.

Demonstrating how visual enthymemes can gain traction and meaning through movement, they argued that "the meanings derived from the placement and display of images in the public sphere come from the experienced contexts in which images have been displayed" (Cos & Martin, 2013, p. 1700). Similarly, I suggest that memes of mental health build in value and create backdrops of shared understandings through their circulation, not because of what is found in them, but because of what is *not* found in them. The in-between premises (the ones derived from contextual knowledges) are the ones that matter most.

Like Cos and Martin's (2013) empty chair, I suggest that the left-out pieces of depression memes make enthymematic arguments about what depression means in contemporary colloquial and medical definitions. Figure 2.1 provides merely one example of a depression meme that utilizes visual enthymeme to make a statement about what depression "looks" like since it may be difficult to explain in words (see Figure 2.1). By using the image of the kitten paired with the caption, the meme in Figure 2.1 jokingly confesses that their mental health is not optimal (the implication is that they have depression). Cats are a popular choice for internet posts in general and memes in particular, so a certain history with cat images is a baseline requirement for understanding.

In the meme in Figure 2.1, the caption reads, "This is what my mental health looks like right now" with a picture of a kitten wrapped in a towel, dripping wet and looking bedraggled, weak, and vaguely annoyed. The meme provides a representation of distress through the illustration of the kitten as unwell, and the viewer is invited to relate to the picture by considering their own state of wellness (or unwellness, as the case may be). By using the image of the kitten paired with the caption, the creator of the meme in Figure 2.1 jokingly confesses that their mental health is less-than-desirable through implicative means—but whether the meme is asking for help, empathy, or pity remains ambivalent.

Cats are a popular choice for internet posts in general and memes in particular. In this meme, the caption reads, "This is what my mental health looks like right now" with a picture of a kitten wrapped in a towel, dripping wet and looking bedraggled. The kitten is being held in a towel and appears weak and vaguely annoyed. The meme provides a representation of distress through the illustration of the kitten as unwell—and yet again leaves open to interpretation how both the poster feels, and the viewer should feel, about this experience of distress. Instead of an empty chair that we are invited to fill in with our beliefs about President Obama (Cos & Martin, 2013), we are presented with a kitten and a caption; in between, we place our own psychological, emotional, embodied, social, historical, and other contextual knowledges to make our own judgment about what it means to be well (or unwell).

Figure 2.1

This Kitten is Not Well

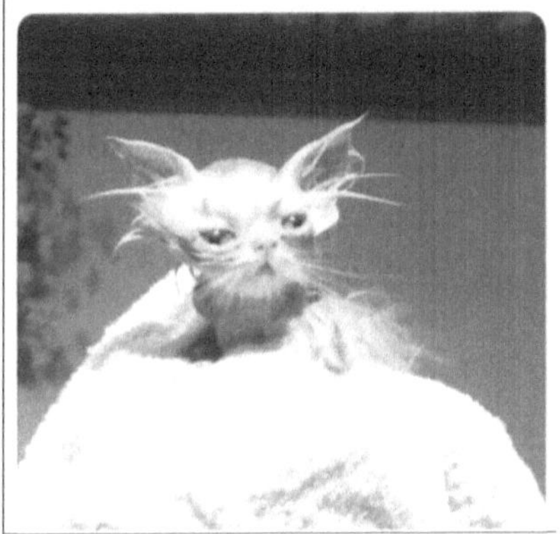

Explicit premises:

1. This is what my mental health looks like right now
2. This kitten is not well

Implicit premises:

1. I am not well
2. To be a mess is to be unwell

This meme is an enthymeme because it operates through a shared recognition of experience. This meme uses an image to describe a person's mental health as dis-ordered through the combination of image and text; neither is sufficient without the other to express the affect suggested by the meme. To understand this meme, a viewer must have a basic knowledge of meme formats; they must have a certain level of experience with mental health as a felt mess. By viewing the kitten's disheveled state, the viewer is expected to relate to the image and recognize the experience of struggling in some way. What the viewer should do with this recognition remains uncertain.

Additionally, memes like this reveal the ineffability of mental illness. Because the meme maker is answering a call to describe what their mental health looks like, this meme confesses a mental health challenge and implicitly comments on the inability to express mental health in another way. The image of the kitten with the caption allows the viewer to *see* what suffering feels like, without cumbersome or lengthy explanations (which may or may not adequately express mental illness' complex realities).

Visual Enthymeme, Visual Memes

While memes are visual texts, the vast majority of memes still use a combination of text and image; that is, image+text here equals a visual assertion of visual and verbal elements. However, these examples show us that even textual memes are visual memes. More to the point, both the more traditional meme combination of image+text and textual memes illustrate that images can be enthymemes through premises delivered by visual means. By asserting that all memes are visual and all memes are enthymemes, I assert that internet memes are visual enthymemes with important ramifications for the study of enthymeme and for discourses of mental health.

Pertinently, scholars of enthymeme debate the nature of the rhetorical text, specifically what counts as an enthymeme: visual or verbal (Lloyd, 2013). Aristotle wrote at a time when the primary format of an enthymeme was oral; later, scholars have mostly focused on written texts as enthymemes. However, recent scholarship has speculated on the visual as enthymematic. For instance, Young (2015) explored the ways that "visual enthymemes function as co-constructed arguments" in a discussion of gendered bodies and the medical gaze (p. 344). Understanding visual texts as enthymeme allows us to view a multiplicity of texts as enthymemes, rather than the traditional "truncated syllogisms" of previous iterations. By freeing the enthymeme from its verbal bounds, we can understand how a variety of texts—including the visual—serve as implicit arguments, which is crucial in a contemporary digital world increasingly flooded with visual texts.

Not all scholars agree, however. For example, Lloyd (2013) urged the need to preserve the "productive and basic oral and written association of the term [enthymeme] that has lasted two thousand years" (p. 747), arguing that using the adjectival form (or, *enthymematic*) prevents a need for settling the debate either way. In Lloyd's (2013) view, the long tradition of considering merely oral and verbal texts as enthymemes is important enough to continue doing so. However, that reason alone seems insufficient. Instead, I assert with Young (2015) and Prenosil (2012) that visual texts can be enthymemes themselves, not merely enthymematic. By making this assertion, I contribute to the growing importance of the visual in rhetorical scholarship, as well as its significance in a contemporary digital culture.

Internet memes are important examples of visual texts because they rely on visual elements for their functioning. While there are some verbal elements in memes, they are delivered to us via visual means and we understand them as having been *seen.* Some scholars have understood memes as combination visual/verbal jokes (for instance, see Dynel, 2016). That is, memes are *both* visual and verbal. However, I next argue that they are primarily visual, as the verbal elements in memes are also visual. Seeing memes as visual (rather than verbal *and* visual) has important implications for visual rhetoric and our contemporary understanding of enthymeme.

Although memes can certainly be heard, watched, spoken, enacted, or lived (as I argued earlier), my primary focus is on memes as *seen.* Visual rhetoric is an increasing area of study in an increasingly visual global cultural sphere. In the past, the study of rhetoric has been focused primarily on verbal texts. However, a rapidly growing area of rhetorical scholarship is noting the significance of the visual in rhetoric (Finnegan & Kang, 2004). Finnegan and Kang (2004) urge a "sighting" of the public sphere, as the study of images "offers possibilities for thematizing vision and images" in a way that "can free us from the impulse to freeze-frame all types of discourse" (p. 396). In other words, exploring images "reveals the need to account for new modalities of public participation" in contemporary life (Hegde, 2010, p. 169). By this view, rhetorical studies should incorporate a view of rhetoric as visual in a global culture that increasingly focuses on visuality.

From a visual rhetoric perspective, visual culture "enables the formation of public discourses and the emergence of publics" (Finnegan & Kang, 2004, p. 394) through shared iconographic understandings. For instance, Olson (2014) explored the circulation of images of the national Ecuadorian identity as shapers and reinforcers of Ecuadorian national pride. Similarly, Hegde (2010) explored the practice of veiled Muslim women in non-Muslim countries and how the veiled female body as an icon circulates as a visual icon of shared understanding. By emphasizing the visuality of memes of wellbeing, I recognize them as circulatory discourses of shared meaning. Understanding memes of wellbeing as visual enthymemes allows us to explore their ability to be tacit, humorous arguments about what it means to suffer in the digital era.

Proponents of purely verbal enthymemes will be quick to point out that most internet memes have text and are therefore not pure images. True, but the premises usually come from the image, or at the very least the combination of image and text. The verbal elements merely set up the joke; both stated and unstated premises come from the images themselves. For example, in Figure 2.2, "Hide the Pain Harold," a popular meme figure, provides the basis of the joke. The text sets up the meme, certainly, but would be meaningless without the image. The text is subsidiary to the image, which provides the crux of the argument and is the memetic, recognizable portion of the meme. Alone, the statement "When someone says, 'Don't be anxious.' And your anxiety is cured" is almost nonsense; paired with the image, it creates a complex, meaningful critique of a social phenomenon.

Figure 2.2

Don't Be Anxious

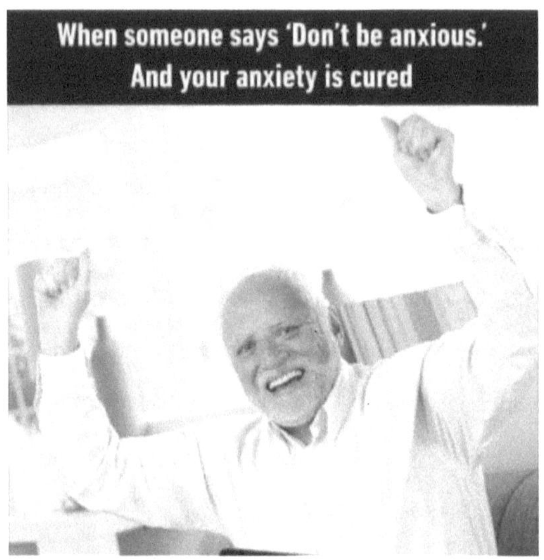

More importantly, the premises of memes come from the *arrangement* of texts. Or, put another way, the visuality of texts creates the argument. For example, in Figures 2.3 and 2.4, there are no "images," per se. However, the memes themselves are screenshots of written posts; they are images of texts deemed worthy of recording (in other words, someone "took a photo" of a text). Moreover, their arguments come from the visuality of the described scene (in the case of Figure 2.3) or the arrangement of the textual elements (in the case of Figure 2.4). Indeed, the popularity of memes that are screenshots of other posts (instead of original image files) underscores the importance of memes as purely visual rhetoric; screen captures of all-text posts (such as in the examples in Figures 2.3-2.4) illustrates that even verbal memes are visual.

Figure 2.3

Everything Is Totally Fine

urbancatfitters

me: [facedown on the floor] listen everything is totally fine

ifunny.co

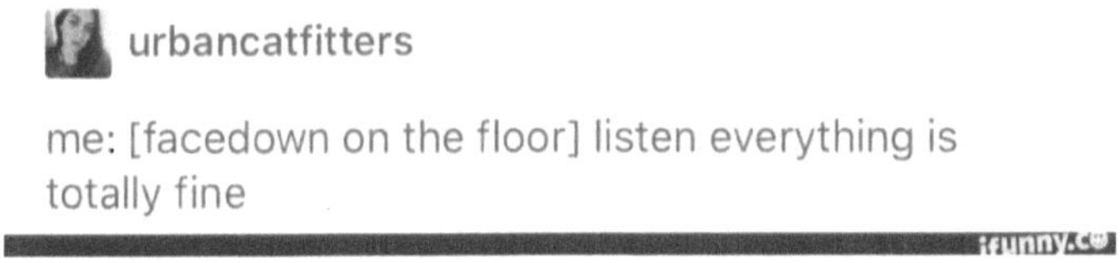

More specifically, the visuality of verbal memes is demonstrated in the ways memes can create visual images with no images at all. For instance, Figure 2.3 is a screen capture of a text post that describes a person "facedown on the floor" and relies on the viewer's imagination to picture the person. Through the text, the viewer is called upon to visualize the person and hear their words as though spoken. This meme, although utilizing verbal elements, is visual in the arrangement of the words, spaces, punctuation, stylization, and other rhetorical techniques; it is further visual because it asks the viewer to *visualize* a depressed person. That is, the audience is invited to see the person lying "facedown on the floor" (an indication of unwellness) insisting that "everything is totally fine" (see Figure 2.3). This is an enthymematic visual depiction of depression because it invites the viewer to fill in the gaps and understand the subject of the meme as depressed, even though there are no "images" in the image (per se).

Figure 2.4

But What If It's Not

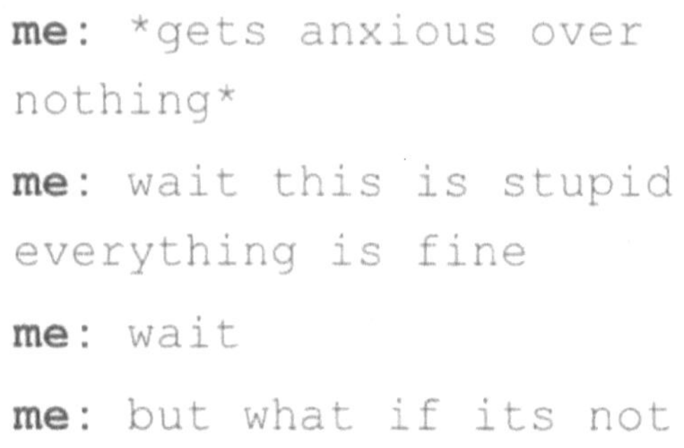

me: *gets anxious over nothing*

me: wait this is stupid everything is fine

me: wait

me: but what if its not

In the case of Figure 2.4, the arrangement of the lines, line spacing, and speech indicators provide the basis for the joke. The spacing of the lines conveys the meaning of time and thought, as the meme depicts a speaker's inner dialogue of suffering. Again, although no image is present, the meme utilizes a particular layout for the verbal elements and subsequent memes captured the screen in such a way as to render this post a meme. Enthymematically, the meme requires a mental visualization of the person (or, more likely, the viewer inserted in the person's place) as the operative step. The audience is invited to see themselves in the shoes of the speaker ("me") and enthymematically visualize themselves in the same symptoms and/or to acknowledge how others experienced these symptoms.

These three example memes are representations of a social experience expressed through a visual joke, rather than a more serious format. Memes, then, as primarily visual forms of rhetoric, can be understood as depictors of abstract concepts; that is, knowledges, beliefs, concepts, cultural tropes, and other taken-for-granted social phenomena are described in memes in unique and particular ways. Gallagher and Zagacki (2007) explored how images make abstract concepts knowable, specifically how "photographs brought what had been previously invisible, in light of the abstract, de-personalized nature of the rhetoric, into clear focus" (p. 125). Similarly, Bacon (2007) noted the power of African American newspaper writers to frame blackness and whiteness in the anti-colonization debate through photographs more clearly than through verbal means. In Gallagher and Zagacki's (2007) and Bacon's (2007) examples, the difficulty of expressing racial tension was in some ways answered by visuality.

In other words, what cannot be easily put into words can be put into images. These images, *in situ*, represent the ambivalent meaning(s) of depression. As these images circulate through a social body, that circulation has important consequences for the social bodies through which they move. As constitutive rhetoric, memes are visual depictions of unknowable experiences of mental health, accomplished through visual representation. Internet users share a collective #mood of suffering through primarily visual enthymemes.

When memes make ineffable feelings or experiences visible, they are working rhetorically in much the same way as other images of advocacy operate. For instance, Gallagher and Zagacki (2007), in an exploration of Civil Rights activism photos in *Life* magazine described photos as "depictions of social experience that are recognizable to common audiences and that add moral import to the decisions or developments before them" (p. 127). That is, images make concrete the abstract and make knowable the unknowable. By drawing attention to "deep rules" in a societal body, visual rhetoric can draw out unspoken concepts and make them understandable in ways not readily expressed (Gallagher & Zagacki, 2007). In the examples in this section, the memers are using visual means to describe what suffering "looks" like, which I explicate further in later chapters. Importantly, the "deep rules" propagate in spheres of circulatory rhetoric, or rhetoric in motion.

Circulatory Spheres

Since ancient times, rhetoric has moved; circulation is thus not a uniquely digital phenomenon (Gries & Brooke, 2018). For instance, Olson (2009) explored the re-circulation of political images during the American Revolutionary War era, noting the "precise relationships" between a body of deliberately similar compositions. Olson analyzed how "compositions were actively engaged and reshaped by the audiences" (p. 6) and how image creators "sought to influence beliefs and actions of their audiences" (p. 6). In Olson's example, political images were re-purposed for particular newspapers' local audiences and the images were later carved into the powder horns of Revolutionary soldiers.

I emphasize historical and physical-world examples as well as digital ones to combat any tendency to think of a meme as a solely ephemeral, internet-era expression. Certainly, the digital age has provided an abundance of opportunity to view and study circulatory rhetoric, but permeable boundaries between digital and physical spaces insist that the demarcation between "online" and "offline" is thin indeed. In another example, Yancey (2018) described QR codes on tombstones, allowing visitors to view memorial websites of deceased loved ones by scanning the link in the cemetery. More importantly, however, Yancey argued that the circulation of tombstones is much older than the web; before digital memorials, family members carved poems, songs, proverbs, scripture, and other circulated rhetoric onto tombstones.

Similarly, memes are known for their movement. Virality is their hallmark; movement is their natural mode of being. To analyze memes as enthymeme is to view them *in situ*, but memes have little meaning if not shared. In fact, they gain their meaning via motion. Circulation studies explores "writing and rhetoric in motion" (Gries & Brooke, 2018, p. 7) to unpack the power of rhetoric as movement. According to the circulatory viewpoint, "rhetoric is all around and within us; it permeates our lives, reassembles collective space, and shapes material reality in all kinds of diverse ways" (Gries, 2013, p. 346). Similarly, Lee and LiPuma (2002) emphasized the cultural power of circulation, focusing on "collective agency and the implications of this performativity for the imagination of social totality" (p. 193). By tracing "the interplay between flows and forms" (Goankar & Povinelli, 2003, p. 388), scholars explore the relationship between both meaning and motion and their cultural consequences.

Circulation theory begins, in part, through the un-binding of the rhetorical situation (Bitzer, 1968). Edbauer (2005) un-frames the rhetorical situation, allowing us to view rhetoric as in flux. Edbauer noted that concept of situation comes from the Latin term *situs,* which "implies a bordered, fixed space-location" (p. 9). In Edbauer's (2005) view, "rhetorical situations involve the amalgamation and mixture of many different events and happenings that are not properly segmented into audience, text or rhetorician" (p. 20). An un-bound rhetorical situation allows us to think of rhetoric as constantly in motion and relieves the tension between the agential audience and rhetor—circulatory rhetoric places agency throughout the circulatory sphere wherein the rhetoric circulates.

Rhetoric on Yancey's (2018) tombstones began elsewhere but ended up carved in stone, ready to be seen by another mourner and used on a future tombstone. In another historical example, Olson (2014) traced historical depictions of the native *rondador* as creators and reinforcers of what it means to be a citizen of Ecuador. The image of the native Ecuadorian, passed through images, narratives, verbal expressions, artefacts, and other rhetorical depictions, circulated and reified the national Ecuadorian identity. The movement of these images through cultural spheres perpetuates certain kinds of meanings as they move.

Affective Representations

While in circulation, depression memes transmit the experience of bodily suffering through visual representations of emotion—or, affect. Affect is the pre-linguistic experience of feelings, or, emotion not yet put into words (Brennan, 2004). Affect studies explores the "something produced through interactions between bodies" (Rice, 2008, p. 211) as an extension of circulation studies. For instance, in a study of affect in internet memes, Jenkins (2016) discussed the way a particular meme "indexes various social attitudes and affections" (p. 463) through its circulation in social networks.

Viewing memes as ambient enthymemes provides a lens to view their emotive power in a contemporary digital sphere, and further allows us to view the emotional, cognitive and embodied aspects of mental health on one plane, rather than dissecting and isolating them from each other. My emphasis on memes as purveyors of embodied emotion is significant; in a contemporary discourse that emphasizes the "mental" in mental health, memers are commenting on the emotive dimensions of suffering and wellbeing.

As a growing field, affect studies provides a useful understanding of the ways "beliefs are constituted through circulating signs and discourses" (Rice, 2008, pp. 204-205). Affect studies often build upon circulation theory to trace the movement of emotion through social bodies. For instance, Brennan (2004) described the transmission of affect as the process by which "the emotions or affects of one person, and the enhancing or depressing energies these affects entail, can enter into another" (p. 3). In Brennan's criticism of psychotherapy, affects literally transfer from person to person through biological mechanisms; for Brennan, affect is the "passage" of emotion through human physicality, carried there by rhetoric. Although affect scholars do not always write of the literal transmission of emotions through biological means (for instance, see Ahmed, 2004), Brennan's understanding of affects as circulatory provides a crucial component for understanding memes as conveyors of an atmosphere of depression.

Figure 2.5

A Long Crying Session

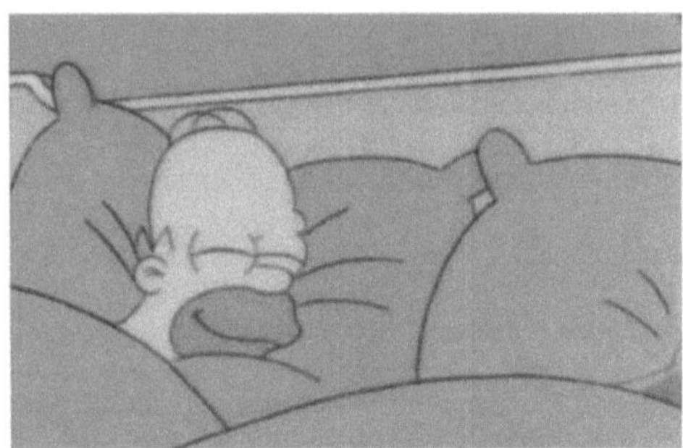

In particular, depression memes require an understanding of what depression means, what it looks like, and, more importantly, what it *feels* like, to get the joke. For instance, Figure 2.4 utilizes a fictional character (from the television series, *The Simpsons*) sleeping with a smile on his face and with the caption, "me after a long crying session finally knocks me out" (see Figure 2.4). To understand this meme, a viewer must understand, at the bare minimum, the experience of crying oneself to sleep; however, the joke is only fully realized when one grasps the personality of the fictional character, the experience of depression symptoms and conventional memeing practices. Importantly, the meme is a depiction of *emotion;* the juxtaposition of sadness and smiling, intensity and tranquility, movement and stillness offer a punchline that self-deprecates and yet glorifies. The meme is funny, and yet it is darkly serious—the proper reaction, after all, is "same." At the same time, a person who does not suffer from depression may connect depression to *The Simpsons*' typical use of humor to debunk or deflate widely shared impressions of public discourses, and to see depression's connection to an animated figure as a trivializing of the illness.

Depression, as an experience, is portrayed in memes that use affective dimensions of rhetoric. Reading between the lines of depression memes reveals an affective stab at expressing the un-expressible; or, making what is ineffable, effable. RQ1 considers the affective dimensions of depression memes and their role as influencers in the experience of depression. That is, depression memes illustrate affects that cannot easily be expressed another way. In Chapter Three, I explore the affective dimensions of depression memes as baseline considerations for a grander project of memes as ambient. Since affect and ambience are inextricably linked, exploring memes as affective expressions is the first step to viewing them in terms of Rickert's (2013) ambience.

Ambience

Combining circulation and affect into ambience provides a lens for viewing memes as a social mood (or, more appropriately, #mood). For Ahmed (2014), "a mood can be what assails from the outside; deciding for us what we can and cannot do" (p. 13). By that definition, "a mood is thus rather like an atmosphere: it is not that we catch a feeling from another person but that we are caught up in feelings that are not our own" (Ahmed, 2014, p. 15). That is, "such a background recedes, or withdraws, even as it generates" (Rickert, 2013, p. 55). Such a view of rhetoric upends the traditional view of agency, as it places agency partly in the hands of the rhetorical landscape. For Rickert (2013):

> ambience itself has a kind of agency, or more precisely, ambience connotes the dispersal and diffusion of agency. While it may not be the agency we customarily attribute to human beings—and while we must grant such agencies different weights and values (which is of itself rhetorical work)—nevertheless, it is of a magnitude and scope to challenge more traditional notions of human agency. (p. 16)

Of course, individuals, groups, objects, technologies, and all other entities within an atmosphere of rhetoric still retain agency, depending on their various "weights and values" (Rickert, 2013); still, providing some measure of agency to the rhetorical ether itself is an important move. Considering collective rhetoric (for instance, memes) as agential allows us to account for complexities in the meanings and scope of rhetorical decisions and outcomes.

So far, I have articulated that circulation plus affect equals atmosphere—an ambient environment of rhetorical *mood* (Ahmed, 2014; Rickert, 2013). In a Heideggerian sense, *Stimmung* (or "attunement" or "mood") is an "already there" embeddedness, or disposition, in the world (Rickert, 2013). By Rickert's logic, rhetoric of all kinds (and, I suggest, including memes) is in relationship with us, and we with it. Quoting Cicero's *De Natura Deorum,* Rickert notes "that not only do we see and hear by means of air, but air itself 'sees and hears with us'" (p. 6). Importantly, "our ambient environment is itself changing; it has accumulated greater conceptual weight and scope alongside the emergence of practices, arts, and sensibilities that are themselves ambient" (Rickert, 2013, p. 9). Viewing memes as air allows us to think of them as rhetorical particles which we "breathe" in and out as both creators and consumers.

Thus, viewing memes as ambient allows us to see them as part of the "air" that we inhale (through rhetorical consumption) and exhale (through rhetorical creation). Like other social moods, the *Stimmung* of sadness "hangs around, despite our best intentions, despite even our own selves" (Ahmed, 2014, p. 13). RQ3 considers depression memes as ambient rhetorical atmospheres. Ambient rhetoric allows a perspective of internet memes as pieces of the cultural atmosphere. This is not to say that one can "catch" depression through memes, per se; rather, the widespread usage of suffering as a trope passes through social bodies and infects the cultural landscape, normalizing depression symptoms and complicating individual and global experience of suffering. While I am not arguing that depression memes *cause* depression (at least, not in the sense of technological determinism), I am suggesting that depression memes reflect and enact a discourse that encourages or promotes suffering in an era that categorizes, labels, and medicalizes suffering-as-symptom.

As I explore the public feeling of depression as addressed through depression memes, I seek, like Edwards (2011), to examine both the meaning and movement of these memes. In particular, Figure 2.5 represents *blockage*: a jumbled mess of bowls in a cabinet, ready to shatter if disturbed. Viewers of the meme are expected to understand the experience of both ineffability and blockage encapsulated by the meme; in other words, the meme seems to say, "we are blocked because we cannot express our experiences and because we are blocked we cannot express our experiences," and so the cycle continues. (Metaphorical) release of the cabinet door would result in disaster, but the sharing of a meme allows the viewer to describe their experience in a way that makes sense to others familiar with memes, depression, and depression memes; it also allows a virtual opening of the cabinet door without any physical-world damage.

Figure 2.6

Let Me Visualize It For You

therapist: you need to open up more

me: i can't

therapist: why not

me: let me visualise it for you

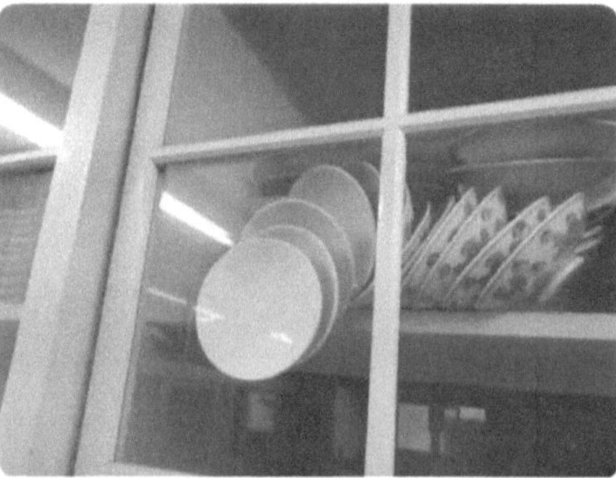

Depression memes' popularity and colloquial depictions as "cures" for depression points to a similar attempt at release through creativity. As enthymematic expressions, they allow users to depict an "in-betweenness" not easily understood, spoken, or relieved. More specifically, depression memes represent the release of cultural blockage surrounding depression, as is neatly summarized by the example in Figure 2.5, which illustrates the ineffability of experience in depression in an enthymematic visualization of, well, visualization. The in-between premises of the bowls-in-a-cabinet meme (a popular mental health meme online) speak to knowledges of depression symptoms, treatment, expression, responsibility, and many other complex factors—all in a few lines and an image. The meme requires a knowledge of depression, coping, and therapy to "get it," and it further requires a mental visualization of what happens when cabinet doors open and glass bowls fall out (along with a mental linkage of that experience with a mental health breakdown).

Circulation, affect, and ambience provide lenses through which to view depression memes as both potentially blockage and release, which, in turn, reflects their ambivalence. Ambient rhetoric relies partly on circulation studies (Rickert, 2013), which addresses Edwards' (2011) concern about both movement and motion and is particularly appropriate for any study of memes and virality. Ambience is also built on affect theory, which considers the circulation of emotion through social bodies. I trace ambience through circulation and affect to lay the groundwork for understanding memes as enthymematic, ambient revealers and doers of depression in our contemporary moment. As these three scholarly areas are so deeply intertwined, a few more words about them here seems appropriate, although I draw upon them separately in succeeding chapters. Ambience is a rhetorical perspective that considers rhetoric as environment; that is, "an ambient rhetoric continually attunes itself both to what is present and to what withdraws: they are the conditions that give rise to our ongoing perceptions and understandings of the world" (Rickert, 2013, p. xiii).

While I discuss these ideas in order, I want to emphasize that each of these rhetorical concepts draws upon the others. In each chapter that follows, I make a case for each through the memes I chose for my sample; although, as I noted previously, the ambient nature of these memes suggests that any categorization is more for practicality than for argumentation, keeping with my project of ambivalence and ambience. The loose categories I use are more for the reader's (and my own) benefit than for any ironclad qualitative analytic methodology, which would too firmly pin each meme into categories (which must be flexible to be meaningful). Both my chosen theoretical lenses and my investigative categories blend and merge in ways reminiscent of my overall topic of ambience; and yet, they are necessary for coherence of study. In the next section, I set forth the research process I took in investigating depression memes.

Investigative Process

Social media discourse has become a significant platform for popular discussions of important topics, including mental health. Some analyses have demonstrated the roles of online forums (such as Reddit or Pinterest) in defining and describing mental health symptoms and interventions (Park et al., 2018; San Jose et al., 2019). A thorough study of depression memes would collect them from all social media platforms, all spoken usage of memes, all material renderings of memes (such as memes printed on office doors or t-shirts), and immeasurable memescape locations, both ephemeral and tangible. As such an analysis would be neither practical nor elegant, I collected memes from a single social media platform: Reddit.

Depression memes lurk in all corners of social media, such as Facebook, Twitter, Instagram, Pinterest, imgur, and other image-sharing platforms; however, I focus on depression memes from Reddit due to their abundance and ubiquity, as well as the sorting algorithms of a platform like Reddit, which allowed me to choose posts by topic, rather than by user, platform, or other distinction. As Reddit memes permeate almost all corners of the web. Reddit is self-styled as "the front page of the internet" (Reddit, 2020), but is more generally known as an originator of social media posts commonly shared in other online spaces, and commonly known as a "dark" side of the internet (rather than anything analogous to a mainstream front page). In particular, Reddit is a popular location for both original and shared memes, as Redditors share their contributions in topical forums known as "sub-Reddits." Sub-Reddits allow users to "up-vote" and "down-vote" favored or un-favored posts, creating a hierarchy of popularity (Shepherd, 2010a; Shepherd, 2020b). Since Reddit organizes posts by topic, all posts on a depression meme sub-Reddit are almost certainly labeled as depression memes by their creators and sharers, although they are also recognizable as such due to their subject matter.

Reddit is a popular platform for meme sharing, and three sub-Reddits will provide my sample: r/depressionmemes, r/depressionmeme, and r/depression_memes. There were four sub-Reddits dedicated to depression memes at the time of collection, but one of them (r/DepressionAndMemes) had only 38 followers, less than ten posts and was designated as a companion to one specific YouTube channel, and therefore too niched for the purposes of research. The rest had thousands of followers (more than 134,000, 180,000 and 134,000, respectively), and hundreds of posts, and were more general in nature. These three sub-Reddits are spaces for sharing memes about mental health, and as such represent a collection of memes that utilize depression symptoms as humor.

These three sub-Reddits are most appropriate for three reasons. First, "depression memes," as defined throughout this book, refers to a sub-set of internet memes that, of course, discuss depression; however, this category is implicit, rather than explicit. That is, to know a depression meme is a depression meme, a user must be "in the know," based on familiarity with the subject matter and internet protocols. Rather than relying on my own subjective understanding of what "counts" as a depression meme, I allowed internet users to make that designation for me. For the purposes of analysis, sub-Reddits using the organizing principle of depression memes as an internet-defined category provide a firmly established sub-set of memes designated by the members of the depression community (rather than relying on scholar-defined interpretations).

Secondly, although I could have searched any number of meme topics on Reddit (e.g., "dank memes," or "memes"), searching for "depression memes" on Reddit provides a broad-enough, but not too-broad, set of memes that encapsulates depression memes as a category. Although search engines, meme sites, and other social media platforms provide countless offerings of memes in the depression meme category (both labeled and un-labeled as such), Reddit (through its topical organization), and these sub-Reddits (through their explicit labeling), provide precise, user-generated meme examples to deepen and strengthen my analysis of depression memes as a category.

Lastly, these three sub-Reddits are most appropriate because the community of users in these three sub-Reddits explicitly designate these memes as depression memes, rather than other mental health diagnoses. Meme sub-Reddits exist for anxiety, mental health, suicide, bipolar disorder, and any number of mental health diagnoses. By focusing on depression memes only, I better aligned my analysis with the topic of post-modern suffering as defined by depression memes, a popularly defined internet category. For instance, had I chosen suicide memes as a topic, I would have failed to incorporate a variety of other depression symptoms commonly discussed in memes, although there certainly would have been plenty of overlap. Indeed, my sample contained multiple memes focusing on suicide, anxiety, and other mental health diagnoses connected with but not strictly regarding depression, further underscoring the need for a precise labeling system for analytical purposes (and suggesting an imprecision of symptomatic labeling in the discourse, as I argue later).

Certainly, some of the memes in these three sub-Reddits use a "darker" shade of humor than can be found elsewhere; some of them are lighter. In many ways, the memes in these sub-Reddits provide a representative sample by incorporating some of the darker memetic tropes alongside some of the more lighthearted ones. Indeed, by providing a somewhat-broad range of examples, these three sub-Reddits best encapsulate the depression meme category. A more exhaustive study of ambience and depression memes would identify thousands of examples from all corners of the internet (and physical-world spaces, too). In the end, I chose to sample depression memes from Reddit because depression meme sub-Reddits provided ready-made repositories of affirmed depression memes (that is, these memes are "out" as memes about depression). A thorough study would have taken thousands of memes from dozens of social media platforms, because depression memes lurk in every corner of the web (as evidenced by my own experience and the additional examples cited throughout my book). However, due to practical reasons and for the sake of (reasonable) brevity, I have chosen memes from three sub-Reddits as handy evidence of the foundations of the depression discourse online.

Significantly, Reddit is colloquially known as a "dark" side of the internet—a place where "edgelords" hang out, even while Reddit memes permeate all corners of the web. Like Tumblr, another popular site known for housing depressed people, Reddit is known to be a place where netizens gather in the wee hours when the "rest" of the world is asleep (although, incidentally, Reddit has some 430 million users as of this writing) (Lin, 2020). Reddit memes end up all over the internet, and memes from other sites end up on Reddit, as Reddit, like any other site, is a collection place for memes. The ebb and flow (or blockage and release) of memes allows for certain gathering spots, although they can be found almost anywhere online.

In subsequent chapters, I use memes collected from my Reddit sample as examples, grouping them into rough categories. However, I emphasize that the loose categories I use for each chapter are not meant to hold meaning beyond simple organization; in order to discuss an ambient, ambivalent discourse in a meaningful way, I had to group them into categories suitable to each chapter for readability and argumentative purposes. These categories are merely waypoints along the ultimate path to ambience, the overarching structure of my book (and the hidden structure of the lifeworld). Each categorical waypoint provides a talking point from which to view and discuss examples of depression in global culture—a thorough reader will easily recognize examples from the ambient lifeworld, not confining themselves to the memes in my sample.

Indeed, my Reddit sample serves the important function of providing ready-made examples of self-styled depression memes to stand alongside a few explanatory examples in each chapter, which serve as points of comparison (and were obtained organically). My interpretation of the ambient lifeworld is heavily clouded by my own experience as a white, middle class, heterosexual, Millennial woman, whose experience with mental health is colored by my rural Southern upbringing, religious traditions, and graduate school education, as well as my part-time job as a Reiki practitioner and meditation coach. As I interact with memes in my own life, I instinctively recognize Reddit memes when enough context is provided, as Reddit is well known for harboring dark memes but differs from other sources (such as Tumblr or Pinterest)—hence, a ready-made source of depression memes less influenced by my own perspective of what entails a depression meme.

To examine the inner workings of the ambient lifeworld of suffering, I needed further specimens to examine which clarified the category of depression memes while maintaining the integrity of the internet-created category, as noted above. I collected the top 25 upvoted posts of all time from the three sub-Reddits during the month of April

2020. This collection period coincided with the beginning of the global pandemic of COVID-19, which provided a unique backdrop from which to explore collective expressions of mental health. At a time filled with uncertainty, tension, and disruption, global conversations about mental health are particularly significant. In beginning of my analysis, I roughly chopped the memes from my sub-Reddit sample (25 from each sub-Reddit, for a total of 75 memes) into three loose categories based on the mechanism they relied most heavily on: To reiterate, these categories are not "hard and fast" designations of what these memes "mean"—they are corrals, so to speak, from which to view them more clearly from the grandstands. Any meme could easily straddle two or more categories, as ambience relies on the permeability of rhetorical thought. My arguments are built on the steppingstones of my own attunement to suffering as a memetic trope; my chosen memes are there to serve as support.

Memes, of course, have logics of their own, and I used my expertise with internet memes as a guide when making these decisions. For the sake of holism, any memes from my sample not utilized as a figure in a chapter have been placed in an appendix for the interested reader (see Appendices). I encourage readers to play and experiment with the categories I chose, because my argument does not depend on the solidity of the categories; rather, it depends on the illumination of the lifeworld as experienced via memes.

Conclusion

Savvy readers will instantly recognize the tropes, practices, and values latent in the memes I use as extant in not only the memes they have personally encountered but also the daily practices of lived experience. Due to my own interests in mental health as a healer and teacher, I view mental health both from a scholarly and personal perspective, as I interact with these memes on a daily basis and discuss them with students, peers, and clients. My experiences as a scholar and participant in the global discourse on depression are colored by these perspectives, which partially align with Cvetkovich's (2012) understanding of activism as a "spiritual" practice as I advocate for mental health sufferers and remedy my own personal attunements toward greater empathy and compassion toward myself and other sufferers of depression symptoms.

In a contemporary culture where jokes influence social opinions, beliefs, and realities, understanding memes as jokes is to understand them in terms of their cultural impact. Current meme studies often focus on political rhetoric, and for good reason (Wiggins, 2019; Woods & Hahner, 2019; Zidjaly, 2017). For scholars of memes and politics, memes represent cultural persuasive tools of activism and social engagement. For instance, Zidjaly (2017) explored how memes "create participatory culture aimed at engaged democracy while saving collective face" for people of the Omani culture (p. 589). Although political rhetoric has global consequences, mental health rhetoric holds significant power for individuals on an increasingly pervasive basis and on an unprecedented scale.

Chapter 3: Visual Suffering

For sale:

Baby shoes.

Never worn.

Supposedly, Ernest Hemingway wrote this six-word short story; however, the concept has been traced to several separate sources in the decades before his supposed authorship and cannot be adequately attributed to Hemingway at all (Budanovic, 2017). Like the frog/joke meme mentioned in Chapter One, the "baby shoes never worn" as a pre-digital meme survives in several different iterations and styles, and now enjoys modest popularity online, including in the meme found in Figure 3.1 and a handful of Tweets, like this one: "For sale. Baby shoes. Never worn. My wife bought the wrong size and they don't fit our baby, who has big feet." (The Devil's own son?, 2020). Another baby shoes Tweet quipped, "For sale; baby shoes, never worn, wife didnt think it was funny to try and put on baby shoes on the cat" (Valdez, 2020). These few variations on one idea bring together several important elements of memeing, including the ambivalent interpretation of an affective story, the interpretation of which relies heavily on the assumed connections of enthymemes, and the ability of memetic practices to wrangle some effability out of complex, ambivalent experience.

Figure 3.1

FOR SALE

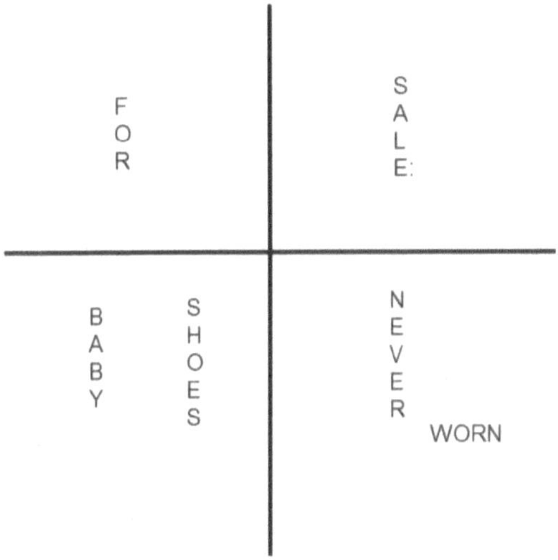

F
O
R

S
A
L
E:

B
A
B
Y

S
H
O
E
S

N
E
V
E
R

WORN

That is, the six-word story about the baby shoes for sale has an affective dimension (sorrow for a potentially dead baby), an enthymematic dimension (as we fill in the spaces between the lines with what must have happened to the baby), and an ambivalent dimension (as multiple interpretations are suggested by the possible enthymematic connections). At the same time, the six-word story eloquently speaks of the complex affective experiences that sixty or even six hundred words might fail to adequately grasp, due to its reliance on the reader to fill in the gaps between the words with their own experience. Depression memes, like the six-word short story about baby shoes, utilize similar in-between affects to create stories of ambivalence surrounding depression. As I demonstrate below, depression memes invite us to participate in a shared, affective space between the spaces of the meme by expressing complex experiential narratives in the space of a few words and an image (or, in the case of some memes, just words or images).

Like Phillips and Milner (2017), I emphasize the complex nature of internet rhetoric, even while asserting my own interpretations of the meaning found there. It is up to the individual reader to determine whether my reading suits their own needs and experience, and how that reading affects their interpretation(s) and experience(s) of dwelling. Throughout this chapter and the chapters that follow, I provide a few potential interpretations of some of the memes in my sample as evidence for the affective dimensions of ambient rhetoric. Like everyone who views a meme, I can merely offer a few potential interpretations and attempt to emphasize their ambivalence as part of a grander ambient lifeworld.

More importantly, the ambivalence of the depression memes in this chapter demonstrates a key phenomenon as part of the ambient rhetoric of depression online. The memes provide half-joking, half-serious depictions of suffering, sometimes couched as depression symptoms and sometimes more generally, but all of them offer multiple meanings of what it means to be depressed. To that end, RQ1 sought to illuminate the affective dimensions of depression memes through an enthymematic lens; by viewing the between-the-lines portion of a meme's message, we may perhaps tease out some of the ambivalent meanings contained therein as part of my larger project to position internet memes as ambient rhetoric. As such, I argue that the memes I explore in this chapter are enthymematic, ambivalent expressions of suffering, sometimes seeking commiseration and other times offering support, although most often doing both simultaneously. Throughout, depression memes offer ambivalent representations of affective suffering.

A Problem with Myriad Names

Depression, as a cluster of symptoms, has enjoyed a controversial history. A variety of labels have been given to a variety of conditions over the past few centuries, including melancholia, neurasthenia, and hypochondria, and more recently depression (Berrios & Marková, 2017; Jackson, 2008; Lawlor, 2012). Feminist literature discusses the relationship with depression to "the problem with no name," as women suffer(ed) the confines of narrow domestic life in changing societal norms (Friedan, 1963; Leissner, 1998), further underscoring the difficulties of describing the varied vicissitudes of a melancholy state. Jackson (2008), in a history of depression's terminology in Western medicine, noted the complexity of depression as a category over the last few millennia:

> As a mood, affect, or emotion, the experience of being melancholy or depressed has probably been as well known to our species as any of the many other human feeling states. The wide range of terms, and the emotional variations to which they have referred, have reflected matters at the very heart of being human: feeling down, blue, or unhappy, being dispirited, discouraged, disappointed, dejected, despondent, melancholy, sad, depressed, or despairing. We have here a range of states that surely touches something from the experience of just about everyone. (p. 443)

While Jackson (2008) notes the ubiquity of the feeling, he also emphasizes the lack of consensus about in medical communities, and at the conclusion of a detailed and complex depiction of the various explanations and treatments for the condition over the centuries, he notes that "the boundaries of what has been diagnosed as melancholia have varied considerably over the centuries" (p. 455), which seems an understatement, given the complexities of the chapter in question.

If the medical community has difficulties diagnosing, labeling, and treating depression, still more so do the individual sufferers of the condition. "Accessing the experience of the depressive in words is, it seems, impossible," as McCulloch (2006) suggested in a study on depressed individuals' connection with poetry and literature to describe their experience (p. 156). Kramer (2006) suggested that "depression lays bare writing's limitations. Words fail" (p. 78). Karp (1994) conducted in-depth interviews with 20 depressed individuals, every single one of whom "described a period of time during which they had no vocabulary for naming their problem" (p. 13).

Depression, both as a generalized diagnosis and as an individual experience, is difficult to describe; it is, in other words, ineffable. Karp (1994) calls this an "inchoate feeling," and noted that "most [interviewees] responded by saying that the feelings were indescribable, but, when pushed to try, they relied on remarkably similar metaphors and similes" (p. 17). The usage of "remarkably similar" descriptions utilizing metaphor and simile is relates to depression memes, which often use figurative expressions in their mechanisms. That the figures of speech were similar further points to an ineffable but shared understanding of what depression feels like.

Another dimension of the inchoate feelings of depression is the complicated decision to "go public" with the information (Karp, 1994; Karp, 2017; Meyer et al., 2016). In Karp's (1994) study, interviewees wrestled internally with whether or not to tell anyone that there was "something wrong" with them, but eventually made the disclosure. Karp (2017) further explored the relationship between depression and identity in a book that chronicles the difficulties of "speaking of sadness," noting that the stigma of depression as an identity creates a dilemma of disclosure. Although online spaces have been known as a place for depression disclosure, talking about depression online is complicated, due to a variety of social factors (Andalibi, Ozturk & Forte, 2017; Corbitt-Hall et al., 2019; Michikyan, 2020).

Since depression and its expressions are so fraught with complications, further exploration is needed to understand its various complexities. Karp (1994) further noted that the "vast bulk of social science research on depression is concerned with establishing its causes and assessing the viability of different interventions for ameliorating or curing it" (p. 8). An example of a social scientific study of this kind can be found in Pratt and Stapelberg (2018), who documented various biochemical and neurological measurements of depression patients as discrete factors as part of an overall project to predict the instance of depression using these factors. If depression is, in part, a sociological problem as well as a biological one (as the literature suggests), studies such as Pratt and Stapelberg's are missing a crucial factor: the affective dimensions of depression.

Affective Enthy-memeing

As noted above, affect studies serves as the first stop on my larger project to establish memes as examples of Rickert's (2013) ambient rhetoric. For a few reasons, affect studies provides crucial underpinnings for the study of ambience (Rickert, 2013). First, affect studies emphasizes the material consequences of emotion, so integral to the ambient workings of rhetorical atmospheres. In Ahmed's (2004b) discussion of "affective economies," she emphasized that "emotions *do things*, and they align individuals with communities — or bodily space with social space — through the very intensity of their attachments" (p. 119). Similarly, memes, as rhetorical carriers of emotion, represent the emotional capital of depression, and an ambient perspective provides a viewpoint of the world as filled with emotional *doings*.

Next, both ambience and affect studies de-emphasize the Cartesian mind-body split as part of a project to de-stigmatize emotion as a driver of human behavior. To that end, Ahmed (2004a) urged "a rethinking of the relation between bodily sensation, emotion and judgement" (p. 5). In a discussion of enthymeme and emotion, Kochin (2009) suggested that the most effective way of gaining one's point is demonstrating that one's argument is self-evident, despite the Western mind's repugnance at emotion trumping rationality. Similarly, I explore how emotion and logic are inextricably linked in rhetorical practice, especially in the liminal spaces of depression memes, which blend the two in intricate and meaningful ways. For instance, Jenkins (2016) discussed the way a particular meme "indexes various social attitudes *and* affections" (p. 463, emphasis mine). Depression memes, in particular, play with cognitive and affective practices.

Lastly, affect studies emphasizes the embodied aspects of emotion. As depression is both mental and emotional, it is also physical—we experience bodily sensations and memes depict those sensations in ways that transcend the human/nonhuman barrier(s). Rickert's (2013) definition of ambience views rhetoric as a conveyance of "our affective investment and emplacement within an environ" (Rickert, 2013, p. 16). Memes represent human bodies, brains, and emotions as in a complex relationship with each other; they are both blockage and release at the points where these elements intersect.

As in the example of the six-word story, the in-betweenness of enthymematic rhetoric is often more important that the explicit portions of the rhetoric; and yet, the in-between hangs upon the guiding structure that holds it up (more on this in following chapters). More importantly, though, the between-the-lines content of enthymemes rely on shared experience and feelings about that experience. The six-word story relies on the reader having some experience with newspaper sales advertisements, baby shoes, and compassion for bereft parenthood if they are to receive the full effect. Of course, a more ambivalent interpretation could take into account sarcasm, irony, ambiguity, and other possibilities of what might have caused the person to sell the shoes. Volumes of fiction could be written on what happened before, during, and after the sale, if someone were feeling curious and had enough time on their hands.

Similarly, depression memes are byte-sized pieces of a grander discourse of what it means to feel in contemporary society, as illustrated by memes functioning as affective enthymemes. In his explication of enthymeme, Walton (2001) argued that the enthymeme functions through the ability of the audience to empathetically place themselves in the shoes of the speaker; that is, acceptance of an enthymematic argument comes as a result of emoting with the rhetor. By that same token, assertions are more persuasive than arguments because to accept or reject factual assertions is to rely on reasonableness, rather than rationality.

Enthymemes work because they ask the audience to give "heightened attention to a contextualized fact and its resultant meaning. The enthymeme is made persuasive not because of the 'piece' that is missing but because of the attention given to it by the speaker" (Fredal, 2018, p. 36). Thus, enthymemes are not intended to persuade through overwhelming force of logic, but rather to induce agreement through shared acceptance of an implicit "bridge" between ideas. The bridging of the gap usually takes place below the surface of conscious thought, and the audience fills in the blanks without realizing they have done so. The enthymeme, then, is an efficient and powerful way to bring an audience to the rhetor's perspective because they will not always be aware that they are being persuaded.

Instead of a linear, rational argument, enthymemes are implicit arguments that rely on intuitive jumps to conclusions, shared between the audience and rhetor. Walton (2001) used the term "plausibility" to replace the term "probability" when discussing enthymeme: in other words, enthymemes constitute what we can reasonably expect to happen, rather than logistically likely. Further, Kochin (2009) differentiated between the "rational" and the "reasonable" to draw distinctions between "argument" and "assertion;" that is, "argument means drawing conclusions from premises that are shared with the audience" (p. 388). By contrast, "assertion means drawing conclusions, or leaving the audience to draw conclusions, from factual assertions that are new to the audience" (Kochin, 2009, p. 388). The six-word story above and the memes below ask their viewers to make similar intuitive jumps via emotional channels, as I demonstrate later on.

Therefore, the emotional component of enthymeme is crucial to our understandings of depression memes. Internet users are sharing in a collective #mood of suffering through enthymemes, which facilitate affective claims through plausible invocations of empathic experience. For Walton (2001), "plausibility is based on something we would nowadays call 'empathy,' the ability to put oneself into a familiar situation in a story or account in which the actions of some protagonist are described" (p. 104). In the case of mental health memes, the affective component is especially important: as sufferers of mental illness describe their symptoms through memetic expressions, they can use enthymematic arguments to represent what is not easily expressed in less complex forms of reasoning. Depression memes, then, require a tacit complicity with suffering through empathy. Enthymemes work because they ask the audience to give "heightened attention" to in-between premises (Fredal, 2018), a notion especially pertinent to ambience and attunement.

Thus, enthymemes are not intended to persuade through overwhelming force of logic, but rather to induce agreement through shared acceptance of an implicit "bridge" between ideas. The bridging of the gap usually takes place below the surface of conscious thought, and the audience fills in the blanks without realizing they have done so. The enthymeme, then, is an efficient and powerful way to bring an audience to the rhetor's perspective because they will not always be aware that they are participating in a particular way of knowing (as Collins suggested in the study about sexism in memes). As such, RQ1 asks how depression memes reveal the affective dimensions of depression, which reveal and do certain kinds of assumptive work about what it means to suffer in post-modernity.

Figure 3.2

PWEEZE

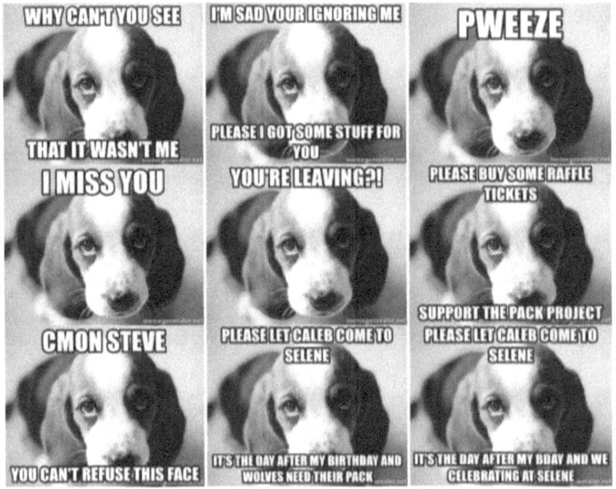

Memes often draw upon emotion for their persuasive power; as a relatively non-ambivalent example, the "sad puppy dog eyes" meme utilizes an image of a begging puppy to persuade its viewer of various requests (see Figure 3.2). Although sad puppy memes can be used ambivalently (often employing sarcasm), by and large, sad puppy memes make simple requests with the straightforward usage of a dog. In some circles, the sad puppy dog meme is known as a "Boomer meme," utilized by an older generation to express relatively un-complicated meanings. Indeed, Millennial and Gen Z memes are known for their increasing complexity and nuance. I include the sad puppy dog meme as a direct contrast to most of the memes in my sample, wherein the affective elements are subtle, implicative, and niched. Generally speaking, however, using *pathos* as a memetic tool is nothing out of the ordinary way of memeing.

Indeed, one of the most common memetic practices is the "reaction image," wherein a statement or caption is "answered" by a visual affective response, such as in the example in Figure 3.3. In reaction images (and GIFs), the picture does the work of a lengthy verbal explanation, standing in as silent communicators of more complex, implicative arguments via affect. In this example, the enthymeme is affective, as emotion stands in for the missing "in between" premises of the meme. Memes, then, invite the viewer to insert their own feelings in the gaps, making a rhetorical "jump" to do so.

Like the examples in the previous chapter, the examples here illustrate that verbal+visual, in memes, corresponds with visual, as the verbal elements become visual in meme images. In Figure 3.3, the subject of the meme "loses" an argument with anxiety, and their reaction is expressed through the image of the young woman whose distress serves as the punchline, though she is not the butt of the joke. The butt of the joke is the invisible speaker, who participates in self-deprecating humor through the affective visual display in the meme. Even the layout of the caption is visual and conveys emotion through the varied capitalization, punctuation, and layout of the two "speakers" in the dialogue. In the end, emotion "wins," as is common with reaction image memes. Most importantly, the in-between premises created by the layout of the verbal elements and their reaction with the image convey ambivalent affects in a variety of meanings and layers. The meme asks the audience to perform a rhetorical leap between the visual elements to fill in the gaps with their own experiences of anxiety and/or their understanding of anxiety.

Figure 3.3

THEY'RE TALKING ABOUT YOU

me: *walks past someone*
person: *laughing*
anxiety: they're talking about u
me: thats not true
anxiety: I SAID THEY'RE TALKING ABOUT YOU

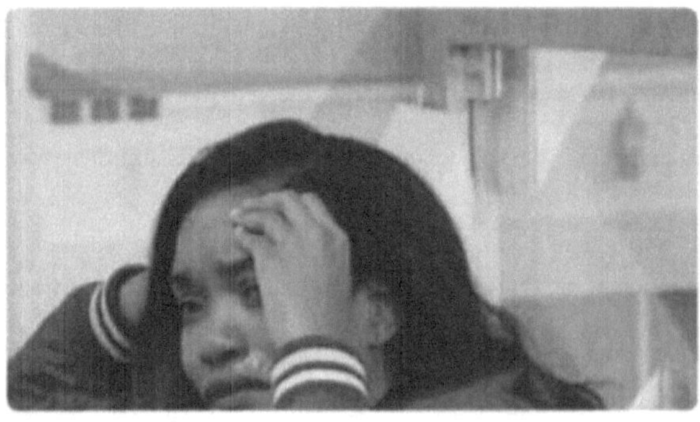

So, memes, as expressions of embodied, ineffable experiences of suffering, are carriers of affective power, hidden in the in-between. If memes carry emotions and these emotions do important rhetorical work, we would be remiss not to understand their significance for depression in contemporary culture. Although I did not include comments in my analysis, depression memes online invite various reactions, from "same," and "mood," to more supportive declarations of solidarity. They may also generate unstated reactions of shock from non-sufferers, who do not see the humor in the meme because they do not draw upon the same set of affects or experiences to make sense of the meme.

The memes in this chapter, then, use affective enthymemes to imply a need for help (i.e., they seem to say, "I have depression") without an open confession of an official diagnosis. Further, depression memes typically have many implied subjects: the viewer, the creator, the sender, and humanity writ large. You, as the subject, are the implied butt of the joke, and you are invited to laugh at your own misery in increasingly complex ways, even while you laugh at the speaker and anyone you might choose to send the meme to. The ambivalent subject implied in the memes further complicates the affect, creating more in-between premises dependent on viewership. The suffering viewer is invited to "fill in" the spaces between the elements with their own affective experience, connecting the loop and releasing with a laugh. This tacit connection creates a picture of what suffering "looks" like through depictions of depression symptoms.

Memes, as enthymematic affective depictions of ineffable experience, do not require complex responses. That is, for those with depression, an appropriate response to these memes seems to be a short laugh and the response, "same!" Although the memes fail to mention depression outright, they depict the symptoms of depression through affective enthymemes, using between-the-lines methods to imply the existence of depression. Depression is the punchline; and the subject of the meme (that is, the person who made it) is the butt of the joke. Through enthymematic expressions of emotion, the viewer is invited to commiserate through laughter in the many experiences of depression, which takes a variety of forms.

The examples that follow provide ambiguous interpretations of what depression "looks" like, affectively speaking, and they do so through ambivalent enthymemes. The in-between premises in these memes invite the subject (an ambivalent Everyperson) to relate to the image by saying "same" (those who experience depression) or "I get it now" (those who do not experience depression). The Everyperson implied by each meme is an affective character that represents sender and viewer alike, but also represents possible others—including those who are being invited to understand the affective dimensions of depression. These collective Everyones are both the joker, the joked-about, and those who may not get the joke. By getting the joke—first of all, "getting" the meme in terms of receiving, participating in online forums, or otherwise participating in it; secondly "getting" the meme by understanding it—the ambivalent subject of the meme complicitly says, "me, too" and/or "See how it feels." The memes in this chapter are divided into three loose sub-categories based on their overarching premises (for more examples of affective memes from the sample, see Appendix A).

What It Looks Like

The first section depicts common experiences of the depressed person through affective, enthymematic depictions of daily life. The two memes in this sub-section (indeed, as in the other memes in this chapter and in the additional memes in the Appendix) illustrate depression memes' ability to make the ineffable effable through the visual depiction of affective suffering via depression symptoms. For instance, the meme in Figure 3.4 explores the complexities of attending a party with depression. In the meme, the subject (an implied Everyman) walks through a doorway into an unseen party, as indicated by the woman standing in the corner (who appears to be talking to someone else just out of the frame) and the usage of the "I'm single and ready to mingle" trope, except that the caption has been hijacked by an alternate caption regarding "joking about my mental health and suicide until everyones[sic] worried" (see Figure 3.4). The meme in Figure 3.4 is also ambivalently self-aware, because the meme acknowledges that joking about mental health and suicide are potentially problematic; the multiple interpretations of the meme provide an ambivalence that implies a mixed support/denunciation of suicide jokes.

Indeed, Figure 3.4 is, in many ways, an anti-joke, although its status as an anti-joke is part of the joke (since its humor is partly due to the expectancy violation of being let down by a not-joke at the end of the sentence). The enthymematic filling up of the room allows the mind to wander through the invisible party attendees, wondering how they might react to such a greeting and imagining oneself in the experience of attending a party with depression. The implication, of course, is that the viewer, spatially positioned as a guest at the party, will commiserate with the sentiment through laughter. The complex experience of carrying one's depression with them into a social gathering (a highly complex and exhausting undertaking) is quickly summed up in the space of one joke; that is, the ineffability of private-depression-in-public materializes between the image and caption.

Figure 3.4

Single And Ready

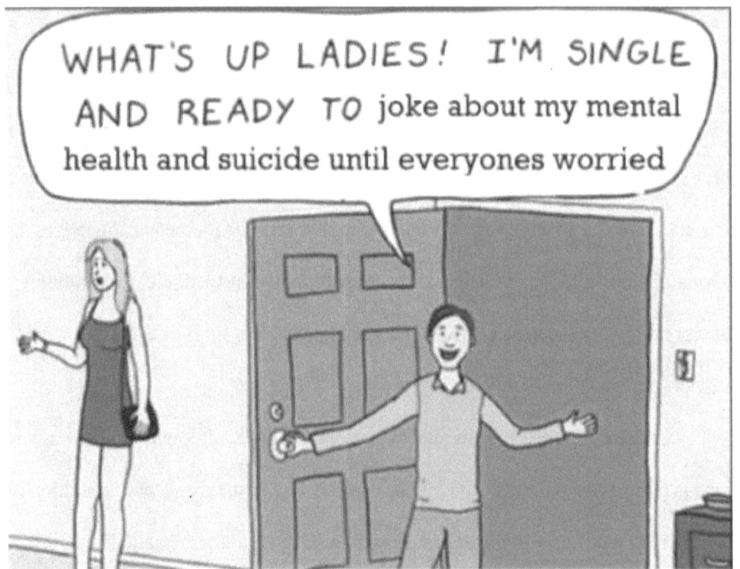

In terms of affect, Figure 3.4 juxtaposes an upbeat party environment with the affects of worry and sadness. Figure 3.4 invites commiseration through a deliberately garbled attempt at ingratiating oneself at a party, which fails in the context of the image but succeeds in the context of the meme. The speaker wears a bright, clean smile and an exclamation point in his declaration, which is, of course, meant to be an upsetting one to the party-goers we cannot see. The humor comes from the jarring switch between the two moods, which nevertheless contains irony—which half of the speech are we expected to connect with the most? The ambivalent emotions push against each other, almost like the implied crowdedness of the almost empty room. All the elements crash on each other with a cacophony that is funny, depending upon one's feelings regarding jokes about suicide and experience of depression symptoms (or lack thereof). Affectively, the meme implies a mixture of feelings that the suffering viewer is expected to share, like the internal turmoil of hiding one's depression from the public eye.

More specifically, Figure 3.4 playfully explores the ineffability of depression through several dimensions, namely the appropriateness of disclosure, the navigations of "out" depression in daily life, and the effectiveness of discussing one's feelings as a coping mechanism. The appropriateness of depression disclosure is explored through the inherent inversion of a party guest abruptly announcing their depression upon entering a room (although, of course, he does not say "I am depressed;" instead, he infers through a memetic trope). Next, the meme takes the viewer through an implied shared experience of navigating a crowded social gathering with depression, leaning into the "cringey-ness" of the experience enthymematically. Lastly, by questioning the appropriateness of outing oneself in a public space, the meme draws on detailed discourses surrounding stigma, disclosure, and discussing one's feelings as therapy—a highly ambivalent experience. The emptiness in the room (which is implied to actually be full) further highlights the enthymemes therein, increasing the ambivalence by allowing the viewer to fill in their own experience. By emphasizing mixed feelings (a party coupled with suffering), the meme draws out an affective experience of individual depression. The meme appears to be a webcomic, so its presence on a sub-Reddit about depression memes indicates a relatability with the sub-Redditors and their experience.

Similarly, Figure 3.5 flips the trend of posting inspirational thoughts online by turning it into a depression joke; although the meme never mentions depression by name, taking the box of a person's "motivation," "will to live," "inspiration," and "happiness" as the objects "you've lost throughout your life" implies that the subject of the meme has depression. This meme (apparently) has two speakers: the first created the inspirational image in the top frame and the second added the sarcastic part in the bottom frame, although both could have been created by the same person (further underscoring the ambivalence in this example). The use of "you" is suggestive, as the viewer is invited into the meme as the person who has lost these things; the bright colors in the top half contrast sharply with the plainness of the box on the bottom, highlighting the emotive contrast between the two spaces. Although the meme uses humor through contrast and ridicule of the first speaker, it also incorporates gallows humor through the choice of objects in the lower box. The ambivalence in the emotive element combines with the enthymeme: “you” have depression (as does the sender, the creator, and potentially others), as well as the mixed emotions between the upper and lower parts of the meme.

Figure 3.5

Things You've Lost

Imagine if someone handed you a box filled with things you've lost throughout your life.
motivation
will to live
inspiration
happiness

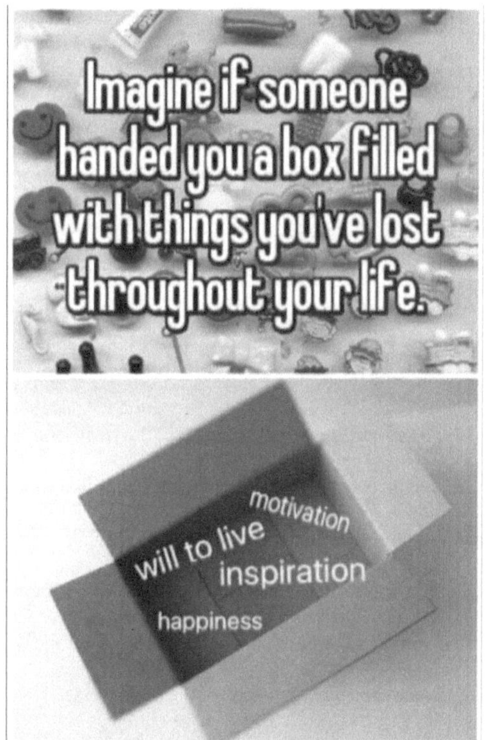

Again, the empty box invites the viewer (an implied Everyone) to fill the box with their own "will to live," "motivation," etc., suggesting that "you've lost" a variety of significant affective objects over the course of daily living. The juxtaposition of "things" (which suggests small, everyday objects), with grander structures (such as "happiness") provides the punchline but also "unpacks" (literally and figuratively) the loss inherent with depression. The experience of loss of appetite, interest, and energy, once commonplace but now missing—or, so the meme implies—succinctly encapsulates a variety of complex symptoms not easily expressed. As feelings are embodied (Ahmed, 2004a, 2004b), the comparison of the objects to feelings is particularly interesting and increases the ambivalence of the meme's structural elements by forcing two opposite ideas within the frame.

The up-ending (literally, one could imagine that the box has been dumped out) of the motivational script, too, questions the viability of hope in suffering in a grimly satirical critique of mental health discourses and motivational culture in general. By asserting the futility of hope, the meme questions the efficacity of belief in a cure for depression, as indicated by the loss of objects not easily retrieved through tangible means. The result is somewhat of an anti-joke, especially since motivational memes such as the top part of the image are common throughout the internet but less common on spaces like Reddit, which tend toward the edgy, dark side of the memeverse.

Treatment

Next, a long-standing ambivalence in mental health discourse can be found in the discussion of treatment: its appropriateness, effectiveness, and who holds the responsibility to seek it. The second category in this chapter deals with the inherent ambivalence in the diagnosis and treatment of depression, which is historically fraught with complication. For example, Figure 3.6 uses a meme format portraying Nancy Pelosi ripping up Donald Trump's speech behind his back, which has been used in a variety of ways online. The example in Figure 3.6 superimposes the caption, "you would feel better if you went to therapy," on the pages of the speech, with the bottom panel showing Pelosi calmly and resolutely ripping it up. Pelosi's ambivalent facial expressions display affectively ambiguous meaning(s), further underscoring the mixed emotions in the meme.

The usage of "feel" better in Figure 3.6 is significant, as "mental" health implies thinking—this meme refers to feelings, rather than thoughts. Still, the deliberate *lack* of emotion on Pelosi's face is in and of itself an emotion and juxtaposes significantly, as a lack of feeling is a symptom of depression. Since the meme is about mental health, it enthymematically implies either a deliberate suppression of emotion or the lack of ability to feel anything at all, and likely includes both simultaneously. The emotions hidden in Pelosi's expression can also be interpreted several ways and could include multiple emotions at once but implies a long-standing personal debate about the merits of therapy. The implication suggests a variety of external and internal discourses summed up in one instant of choosing to tear up a piece of paper.

Figure 3.6

You Would Feel Better

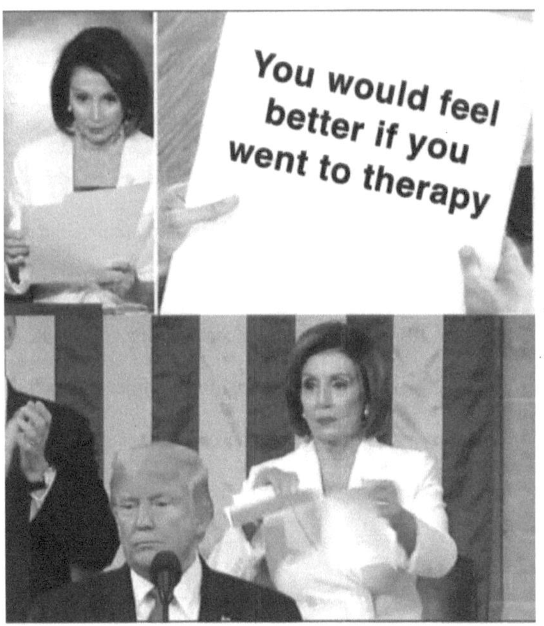

Depending on a viewer's political opinions, experiences with therapy, and a variety of other factors, a viewer could infer a variety of meanings from the in-between spaces of the meme in Figure 3.6; however, overall, it seems to invite laughter and connection over the need for therapy, even while contradicting the value of therapy. The idea(s) contained on the paper exist at the center of ambivalence(s) that tease out a number of significant depression discourses. Indeed, an ambivalent reading of this meme emphasizes conflicting emotions about the validity of therapy, the agency of mentally ill persons, implied familiarity with this same internal debate, and other emotive experiences, held simultaneously and in contrast to one another.

Using enthymeme, the meme converges therapy, mental health, and humor in an ambivalent participation in mental health discourse. By inviting commiseration with implied depression, the preceding examples use affective enthymematic expressions to comment on the experience of depression through humor, and they do so in a way that captures (or attempts to capture) the ambivalent, multi-faceted experience of depression through self-deprecating laughter. By implying that both the meme-maker and the viewer are butts of the same joke (depression), these memes create affective connections between those who share them.

Affectively, the meme in Figure 3.7 uses a variety of fear-based emotions, and then invites us to laugh at ourselves and the experience of medication that seems to have no effect whatsoever. The meme utilizes implicative graveyard humor to carry the reader's eye from the sinister image at the top down the page to the line drawing beneath. The viewer is further invited to experience themselves in the childishly-drawn wolf down below, even as they are invited to understand depression on medication as only a slightly-younger-version of depression itself. The meme invites us to feel a variety of ambivalent emotions on behalf of the meme's subject, whose presence seems less immediate than the memes in the previous section; the juxtaposition of grim, dark affects in the top panel further the book when placed alongside the release of fear through the childlike drawing in the panel below.

Figure 3.7

Depression With Medication

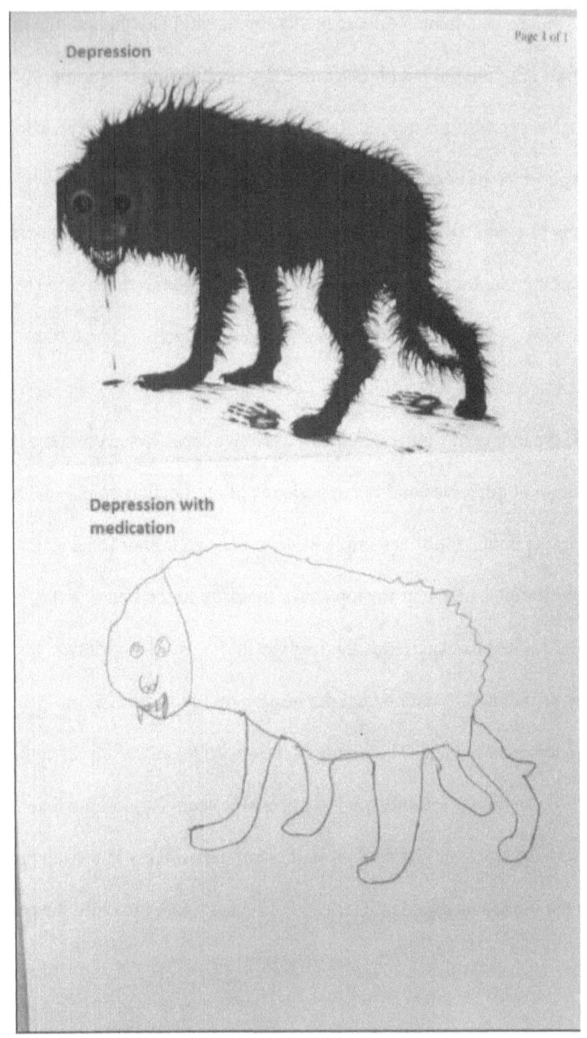

The meme in Figure 3.7 proposes a variety of implicative suggestions by combining the cognitive associations of medication, horror fiction, and artistic precision with the affective elements of fear, childishness, and doubts about medication's effectiveness. These implicative suggestions depend largely on the viewer's experiences, including their relationship with the sender, along with their previous experience of memes of this type. However, the choice of a wolf to represent depression speaks to the embodied aspects of affect; the animal nature of the wolf serves as a contrast to the human images in other depression memes. As an animal form of human nature, depression (in the form of the wolf) seems to represent a non-human element to depression, a suffering that can only barely be controlled (even by medication).

Cultural nuances about the character of wolves, too, serve as an additional ambivalence, depending on the viewer's own schema, and are likely aligned with Reddit's tendency toward edgy, dark humor. As merely one example, the most obvious dimension—that of the effectiveness of medication—is played out in the contrast between the two pictures. The embodiment of depression as a "wolf" (an enemy to be feared) and then a "tamed" version of the same animal is an interesting implicative choice; it suggests ambivalently that depression on medication is still, after all, depression. The meme's two images provide a depth of expression and nuance through their contrasting images and the space between them, encompassing a vast discourse about medication and the passage of time. This passage of time, though present throughout this chapter, is further highlighted in the memes in the following section.

Charting Growth

A final connecting thread in this chapter is the idea of growth (and/or the lack thereof) through depression. For instance, Figure 3.8 uses Will Smith, a popular meme figure, alongside Marylin Manson, who also appears in a variety of internet memes (many of them about depression, incidentally). The image of Will Smith next to Marylin Manson has been memed several times, as the obvious juxtaposition readily steps in to serve as a punchline. In this example, however, the gap between Manson and Smith seems to be filled in with coming-of-age: between "teen" and "thirties," it seems, one could infer years of struggle, diagnosis, coping, medication, and any other relevant experiences that the viewer chooses to fill in.

Affectively speaking, this meme is almost two reaction images in one, as each face draws the viewer into separate experiences of youth and age. More importantly, this meme spans years of realization, ineffability, and growth in the space of a single picture and a few captions. The period of time spoken of by Karp (1994; 2017) as inexpressible seems to hover like a phantom, just between the two figures, expressing a narrative of emotion not easily expressed even in a novel-length coming-of-age story. This gap stands as an enthymeme in its own right, as the viewer is invited to fill in that gap with the years of their own life, using "dark" as a general reference to clothing, demeanor, behavior, and, apparently, depression (especially appropriate on Reddit, which is known for "dark" humor). The implicit need to "show the world" hangs over the entire scene like a haze, further pointing to the ineffability of depression coupled with an unshakeable urge to somehow describe it despite our insufficiency to do so.

Figure 3.8

Showing the World

me in my teens
showing the
world how
dark I am
me in my
thirties, way
darker
but dressing
comfortably

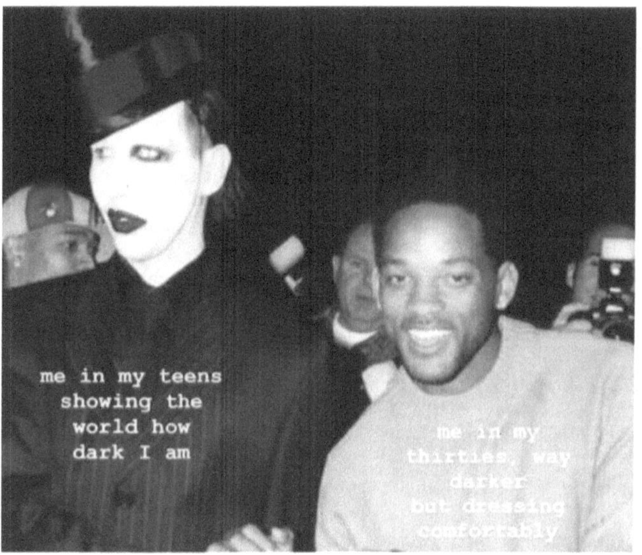

Further, ambivalence is the heart of the meme in Figure 3.8; the expression on Will Smith's face can be read a variety of ways (ironically, sincerely, and sarcastically, just to name a few), and the gap between them can be filled in with individual experience. As an enthymeme, the meme invites commiseration with depression without ever mentioning a single symptom beyond "dark," and "darker;" the implication is that the "phase" of the teen was merely an early expression of what would turn out to be depression. The ambivalence, too, comes from the connection of the various elements of the meme, as facial expressions are read to be as both "happy" and "sad," or rather that

Manson and Smith are putting on a particular face for the camera while hiding an inner turmoil. A strained smile is a meme in its own right, and occurs in many depression memes, so its usage is particularly appropriate in a meme that represents the navigation of childhood-to-adulthood through depression.

Even the interpretation of "darkness" in the image provides an ambivalent reading, accentuated by the darkness of the background contrasted with the flashbulb camera (although this element is certainly more subconscious than deliberate). The visibly "dark" figure of Manson staring offscreen, contrasted with the verbally "darker" (in itself a racially charged joke) image of Smith, underscores a layered interpretation of darkness. Skin color adds a further layer of nuance, as Smith is literally "dark" (see Figure 3.8) and Manson's face is painted white—a play on authenticity and self-hood. By visually distancing the viewer from the younger self (as represented by Manson looking off-frame) and connecting the viewer to the adult self (as represented by Smith's direct-angle view into the eyes of the viewer) the meme suggests an emotionally complex self-as-depressed. Never mentioning depression by name but eloquently describing an ineffable passage of time (imbued with development and growth), the meme enthymematically illustrates years-worth of ambivalence in one short joke.

Similarly, Figure 3.9 implies *impatience* through its injunction to have "patience" (see Figure 3.9). The meme makes no pretense at humor, although a grim irony can be derived from the many-layered elements the man is tangled into. This meme openly calls for support through a relatively un-ambiguous expression of struggle; however, ambivalence remains firmly in the mix when we consider the dark satire found in the figure watering the tree that will ultimately raise the noose around his neck. The tangled elements imply frustration, contrasted with the suggestion of "patience" at the top; in between the lines is a suggestion of depression, with all its difficulties and struggles. Although depression is never mentioned, the meme ambivalently implies both healing and suicide, juxtaposed in a meme that invites social support through its suggestiveness. By suggesting that the viewer relates to the experience within, the meme invites the viewer to experience depression with the meme's implied subject.

Even the blank spaces in the image itself seem to invoke a contradictory emptiness/fulness, as they speak to the complexities of speaking out about depression simultaneous to coping with day-to-day life. The empty space around the figure and between it and the word "patience" underscore the enthymeme here, as the viewer is invited to fill in that space with their own experiences and understandings of emotional experience. The lone verbal element is also a visual one, as its stylized placement contributes to the mood of the image. The lone figure seems to represent an Everyman (or, perhaps, Everyperson) who colludes under a collective injunction toward patience but ultimately does so alone, and, by so doing, waters the trunk of his own noose.

Visually, the meme in Figure 3.9 is a complex discussion of the nature of care. By focusing on the visual elements alone, we follow a cyclical exploration of growth; self-care (as implied by the man watering the plant) is a form of healing that simultaneously promotes death. The fist-like grasp of the other end of the noose intertwined with the watering can, limbs of the plant, and the figure itself represent a complexity not easily expressed verbally. However, the verbal/visual element—"patience"—implies a further ambivalence. Who is suggesting the patience? Is it supportive? Or commanding? In many ways, it is both/and, further underscoring the complexity of depression as an affective experience.

Figure 3.9

Patience

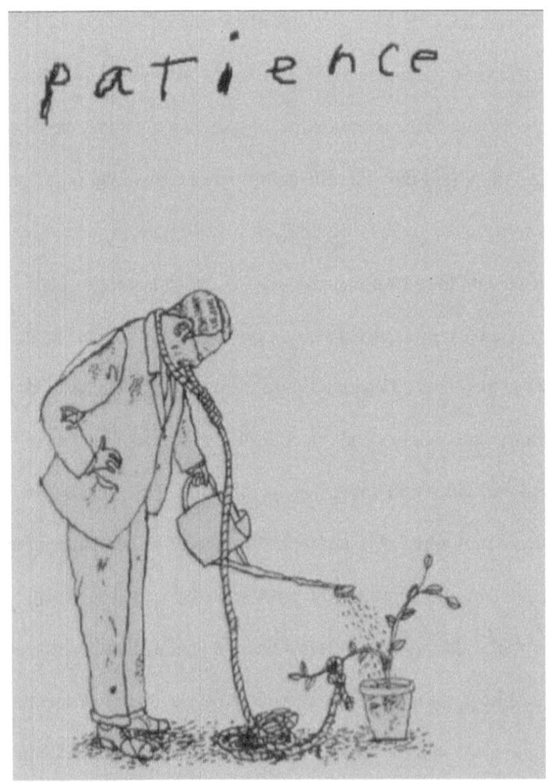

In these final two examples, growth is portrayed ambivalently as inevitable but carrying a mixed bag of mixed feelings. Growth, here, suggests an ability to view depression differently, and yet an inability to escape its confines. Growth in and of itself is portrayed as both desirable and undesirable, as something to be sought after, but by whom and for whom? The examples in this chapter draw upon affective enthymemes to explore what it means to be a depressed person, and by extension, what it means to be Everyperson. The ambivalent self/other, via enthymeme, stands in for other memers, including the viewer and possible other selves. Affect, here, invites *you* (and me, and anyone else who sees the meme), to place ourselves in the shoes of everyone else. Overall, the memes in this chapter invite ambiguous affective connection through bids for both commiseration and support.

The affects of depression featured in the memes in this chapter "reveal" ambivalent interpretations of what it means to experience depression symptoms. As a largely ineffable, indefinable experience, depression demands highly nuanced tellings. Alongside the centuries-long definitional project of depression, memes stand as minute testaments to the impossibility of putting suffering into words. For sufferers of depression, viewing a meme that succinctly and authentically captures the affective dimensions of suffering through the spaces "in-between" effability, affective enthymemes provide a brief moment of "same" as they recognize the punchline. Further, the small instant of chaos (*zhama*) through laughter releases the blockage (*hisa*) of ineffability (Edwards, 2011), reminiscent of Cvetkovich's (2012) suggestion of release through creative expression (which I discuss more later).

Notably, every example in this chapter included an implied subject—the invisible subject of the meme (perhaps representing sender, receiver, or someone else) who is invited to have depression with the invisible rhetor. Memes are largely anonymous; even if the original poster is included, they are rarely known as the creator of individual memes (that is, memes are usually not "signed" like artwork, even if famous meme-makers carry a characteristic style—although some meme-makers will use their semi-anonymous usernames as signatures). As such, the invisible subject of these memes is an indefinite Everyman (or Everyperson, or Everyone) who is invited to take turns being the subject of the meme as the meme passes from viewer to viewer. This Everyperson invites complicity with suffering through the exploration of depression, which memes "reveal and do" (Rickert, 2013) through their affective elements. The enthymematic presence of the invisible Everyperson suggests an ambivalent connection to the affect of suffering, along with a contrast between the individual sufferer and the public experience of "out" depression.

As enthymemes, these examples persuade us into various interpretations through "reading between the lines" of affective connection. These memes persuade through enthymeme, as they take for granted certain assumptions as their initial premises. More plainly, depression memes seem to vacillate between "I need help," and "I'm okay!" almost like a hurried, shuffling request for assistance followed by a quick, "jk!" (I am forcibly reminded of two youngsters from Verona, who insisted that they do not bite their thumb at *you,* sir…but they *do* bite their thumb, sir, just in case you might notice). Each of these memes hide the message in the empty space *between* the message, which is much more complex than first meets the eye. Alongside the complexities of disclosure, memes stand as an interesting way to "out" oneself as depressed through the half-joking, half-serious ambivalence the internet affords.

Conclusion

Both enthymeme and affect provide rhetorical lenses that call for a minimization of the mind-body split (affect does so for obvious reasons, enthymeme for more subtle reasons, which I outlined in this section). Rather than decocting, analyzing, and objectifying the human experience of depression as a purely cognitive experience, I emphasize the affective elements of mental health through memes that explore both the cognitive and emotive dimensions of depression. This is in line with Rickert's (2013) assertion that "affectability is lived in the attunements that illuminate our being-together-in-the-world. The world, as both matter and meaning, is inseparable from how we are and what we do" (p. 15). The memes in this chapter seem to echo this charge, as they focus on the affective, embodied aspects of depression as something ineffably embodied; felt, rather than sensed. By inviting the viewer into that same lived experience through affective enthymeme, these memes invite the invisible Everyperson into affective knowledge of the experience of depression.

Chapter 4: Baggage

"Cursed" images are internet pictures tainted by a vague sense of wrongness or evil, and they circulate as morbid jokes. According to the meme tracking site Know Your Meme, cursed images are "generally pictures or photographs that are seen as disturbing to the viewer, either due to the poor photo quality or content within the image that is abnormal or illogical" (Cursed Image, 2020). More simply, cursed images are the meme-sized version of a horror film; typically, they draw upon disturbance and curiosity as their source of entertainment. Cursed images are merely one example of internet culture that dwells in the dark and dismal, and they do so through the circulatory nature of online spaces. Because memes provide a framework for knowing the world, understanding individual *topoi* (such as memes) can point out our "collective consciousness" (Czyzewski, 2001), or what internet users might refer to as "#mood." As ambivalent internet rhetoric, the cursed image is both popular and cringe-worthy, scary and cool, good and bad, funny and creepy all at once; this insider knowledge is produced through familiarity via circulation. They operate from shared ontology—as do depression memes.

The cursed image, like the depression meme, implies circulatory in-groups and out-groups online which, through enthymematic leaps, invites the viewer to join a "club" of like-minded peers. Like Edwards' (2011) *hisa* and *zhama,* the conglomeration, stagnation, release, and flow of images online operate through motion. That is, the motion of images represents a physical leap coupled with the enthymematic leap between ideas that only users familiar with the tropes will understand.

In particular, *topoi,* as one of the oldest forms of circulatory rhetoric in Communication literature, provide a parallel example of how memes circulate in a discursive body. Although Rickert's (2013) understanding of ambience focused on *topoi* more generally, mostly referring to them in connection with the *chora* (which I discuss later), more discussion of the *topos* is needed here, due to its relationship with both meme and enthymeme. As an example of a relevant *topos*, to know an image is "cursed" requires an enthymematic understanding of internet spaces; one must "fill in the gaps" between discourses, *topoi*, and rhetorical practice when making these kinds of rhetorical jumps. Similarly, depression memes require insider knowledge of various topoi in the circulatory spheres they inhabit.

Cursed

The visual form of creepypasta (the social media equivalent of a horror film), cursed images constitute a circulatory mood of fear, appearing on various platforms and using variations of the same theme of disturbia in its variations. To know that an image is cursed, you must be deeply entrenched in the internet culture(s) that produced it. The photo itself is, in turn, deeply entrenched in that same culture, as the cultures are (more or less) entrenched in each other. Although cursed images are often labeled as such, the cursedness of the picture is evident to those in their circulatory realm. To be cursed, an image must not merely be terrifying. Cleanly edited or finely polished horror material is not cursed (for instance, a professional image taken from a horror film is not cursed, merely scary); a "cursed" image must also be a lo-fi picture shrouded in mystery, with an air of home-video user-generation. Internet users know a cursed image when they see one, due to the circulatory nature of the practice. Because these images have circulated on so many platforms, to see a cursed image is to know that it is cursed by its embeddedness in a variety of interconnected discourses.

For example, Figure 4.1 (a cursed image from a web search) utilizes fear, aggression, and intimidation in the layout of the various elements, the topic of the photo itself, and the editing of the photo's filters and lighting. At the same time, a cursed image is ambivalent, as any viewer could argue for or against its level of cursedness, or even rank a series of pictures according to the amount of cursedness contained therein and must hold multiple dimensions of (positive and negative) emotion in mind while viewing the picture. Knowing when an image is cursed or not (or how cursed the image is) requires rhetorical attunement to the *topos* of cursed images online through familiarity with cursed images and online practice. The circulation of cursed images illustrates the power of internet rhetoric to create inclusion through exclusion. By posting images that are repugnant to those not "in the know," cursed images create an in-group of those who "get it" by excluding anyone who does not.

Thus, cursed images are a different kind of affective enthymeme; they require hidden premises surrounding emotional knowledge, but they do so in circulatory spheres. Depression memes, similarly, require emotional knowledge (or, one could say, "baggage") to make leaps through circulatory structures. In other words, affective enthymeme combined with circulation allows us to view not only the in-between premises between individual meme elements (meaning) but the in-between premises between memes, discourses, cultural objects, meme structures, and other rhetorical objects (motion) (Edwards, 2011). The enthymematic leap here is not between emotional elements of the meme but through the circulatory structures of memetic *topoi* online.

Figure 4.1

A Cursed Image

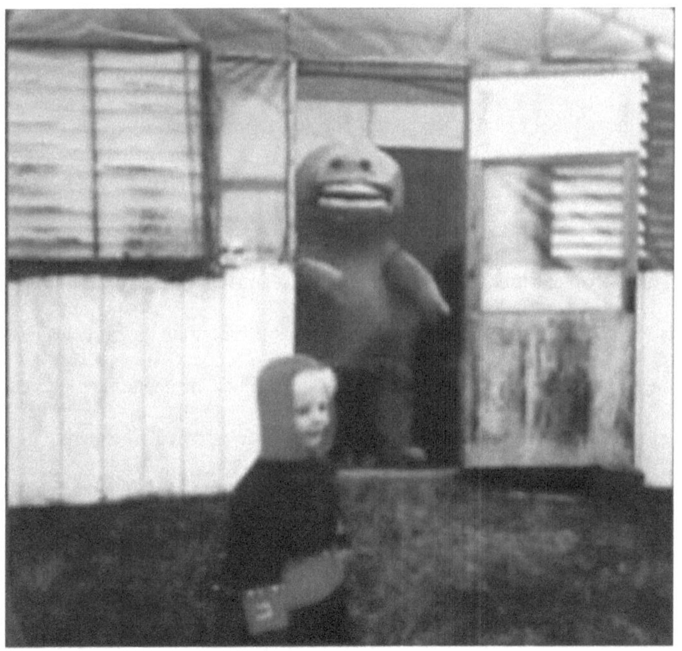

As such, depression memes represent an ambivalent and complex interpretation of circulatory depression; my interpretation merely takes a few of the possible interpretations into account. In this chapter, I make two distinct yet intertwined arguments. First, I argue that the *topos* of depression is deeply embedded in the circulatory cultures of the internet, and that internet cultures are deeply embedded in circulatory cultures of depression, both challenging and perpetuating a circulatory attunement toward suffering. Second, I trace a few *topoi* found in depression memes, which illustrate the threads of depression woven through our post-modern discursive tapestry as examples of how the *topos* of depression figures in online discourse. That is, I first discuss depression as a topos found online and then provide a few examples of specific memetic topoi found in depression memes. Overall, depression memes as circulatory, affective enthymemes allow the Everyperson to participate in collective "baggage" as they interact with memes online.

As in Chapter Three, the *topoi* of depression and depression memes in this chapter are both/and. Significantly, in this chapter, the Everyperson from the previous chapter places the emphasis on "every" instead of "person"—since the memes are in circulation, they are in partnership with others joining in on the joke. Although the memes in the last chapter contains elements of connectivity, the memes in this chapter underscore the collective nature of suffering, whether precisely identified as clinical depression or more generally labeled as a vague kind of post-modern suffering. These memes, via circulation, demonstrate a keen awareness of themselves in relation to others, implying through enthymematic leaps that everyone is in on the shared "joke" of depression symptoms. As circulation theory is a crucial component of ambient rhetoric, by coupling it with the affective dimensions of memes, a picture of depression emerges that illustrates the circulatory power of rhetoric. The usage of "everyone" in depression memes suggests a circulatory "club" of suffering persons joining in collective humor.

Importantly, though, not everyone is in on the joke; some of the memes may produce discomfort among those who do not suffer from depression, as a major purpose of these memes is to connect with like-minded others in depression circles online by identifying those who fail to be shocked by the image. In the same way that cursed images cause inclusion through exclusion, depression memes in this chapter use a debonair grimness that identifies members of an online "club" of depressed people. Simultaneously, though, the enthymematic circulation of depression memeing is ambivalent; even while their circulation creates exclusion through dark humor, they also create inclusion through affective connection (as described in the last chapter). The resulting discourse is one of mixed emotional circulation, as depression itself (in its nebulous "we are suffering" form) circulates online.

As such, one way to view memes as circulatory objects is through the classical rhetorical concept of the topics (*topos*). Aristotle's *topos* has usually been translated as "commonplace" (Dyck, 2002). Jansen (2007) provides an "untimely review" of Aristotle's *Categories* in order to explore its relevance in the contemporary information age. In an era when information abounds, computer systems must organize, categorize, and label the vast quantities of research that are produced every single day. Similarly, Said and Silbey (2018) analyzed digital age *topoi* to demonstrate the ways that "narrative *topoi* live in contemporary popular culture" (p. 104). Though an ancient concept, *topoi* survive as ways of explaining tropes or themes in digital society; if we can understand internet memes as commonplaces, we can categorize and understand them as Aristotle did.

Indeed, *topos* and enthymeme have been closely linked in scholarly work, as Dyck (2002) argued that the *topos* is a binary relation which contributes to an enthymeme, although many modern readers confusedly believe they are one and the same. By unpacking the *topos* and the enthymeme, Dyck argued that enthymemes consistently "substitute another relation, a *topos*, for the relation of implication as they move from syllogism to enthymeme" (p. 111). For my purposes, linking *topos* with enthymeme provides an important connection; understanding memes as commonplace enthymemes allows us to think about them as implicative arguments through shared cultural meanings.

Viewing the enthymematic qualities of internet memes grows important when we consider the implicative power of digital *topoi* in the form of internet memes. The images in the previous chapter on affect utilized depression mostly *in situ*; that is, they discussed depression from a (relatively) static viewpoint. Memes, however, are known for their circulation, and the memes in this chapter emphasize circulatory spheres. RQ2 inquires of depression memes and their tendency to pass on digital *topoi* of and about depression. Although all memes are by nature circulatory, in this chapter circulation takes on multiple layers of meaning. Like the six-word stories of the previous chapter, circulatory memes provide succinct, affective snippets of knowledge about what it means to be depressed, but with the added element of motion. Motion, after all, is how memes make their claims.

Having analyzed depression memes for their affective qualities, their circulatory qualities now take center stage; this chapter discusses depression memes as powered by movement. The memes in this chapter are the memes from my sample that spoke the most of movement. I selected them because their message relied more heavily on movement than otherwise; indeed, the movement *is* the message. I organized them loosely by topic; however, as with all internet rhetoric, their ambivalence keeps the boundaries permeable. In this chapter, I describe four specific topics as illustrations of the threads of depression woven through the generalized tapestry of suffering, although these four are in no way representative of the whole. Suffering, as a *topos*, contains many other topics online, and these four common examples illustrate the many flavors of depression memes.

Rhetoric in motion

Although memes are known for their circulation, they are not unique in doing so. In Yancey's (2018) example of tombstones and circulatory rhetoric, rhetoric moved from stone to digital code and back again as part of a broader circulation of online and offline discourse. However, the tombstones illustrated circulatory practice even before the QR codes were added; epitaphs and grave labelling practices circulated centuries before the invention of the internet. Rickert (2013) further notes the Latin roots of the word "ambience," which designate a "going about"—further underscoring its connection to circulation (p. 5). Indeed, "rhetoricity is the always ongoing disclosure of the world shifting our manner of being in that world so as to call for some response or action" (Rickert, 2013, p. xii). In other words, ambient rhetoric "surrounds; it is of the earth"

(Rickert, 2013, p. x), and illustrates "a fundamental reciprocity between world and person" (p. 6). To view the world as ambient, we must first view it as a locale of circulation.

As noted previously, circulation theory establishes rhetoric as motion. Visual rhetoric, in particular, serves as an example of rhetoric that moves from digital to physical and back again, building upon itself as it mixes and mingles with other rhetorics nearby. Indeed, images "undergo mass (re)composition, (re)production, and (re)distribution and rearrange collective life" (Gries, 2013, p. 336). Yancey's example of the QR codes on tombstones ties particularly well to ambient rhetoric, which Rickert (2013) argued "surrounds us as material, spatial, and environmental" rhetoric (p. 16). From a circulation perspective, the movement of rhetoric provides meaning beyond the meaning of the object in its stationary form. Scholars concerned with the constitutive nature of rhetoric argue for the power of images as binders of social groups; indeed, "society is possible because of the binding forces of shared information circulating in an organic system" (Carey, 2009, p. 7).

As images circulate through a social body, that circulation has important consequences for the social bodies through which they move. Memes, in particular, grow in complexity and nuance through time, as the originator of a meme utilizes previous memes, outside knowledge, combinations of multiple memes or cultural references, and other multi-layered elements to compose further memes. That is, if a user sets out to create a new meme, they will draw upon previous iterations of that meme genre and add layers of image or text to create a more intricate meme than previous versions. Like a variation on a theme in jazz improvisation, memes become more obscure (colloquially referred to as "dank") as they travel through internet spaces. The niche aspect of memes is important, as the implicative layers added with each new rendition create new meanings that have different cultural meanings in different contexts. Thus, meme viewers must be familiar with a variety of outside knowledges in order to understand more obscure specimens.

In this chapter, I focus on the circulatory nature of memes of depression, emphasizing their position in a network of moving parts. Depression memes move through a multi-layered environment of information about what it means to be depressed, and they draw upon meme culture, mental health rhetoric, and a variety of cultural tropes to do so. Thinking of depression memes as enthymematic *topoi* provides a lens through which to see depression memes as molecules in an atmosphere of mental health discourse. In Olson's (2014) work on indigeneity and narrative imagination, she argued that "the familiar can serve a generative purpose" through the repetition of recognizable ideas (p. 7). Olson viewed *topoi* as inherently persuasive; that is, "places of return in changing circumstances that allow rhetors to make claims both on and from within" (p. 5). In other words, users both within and without a culture might view tropes as identity markers that affirm and re-affirm particular identities.

In a similar manner, memes function as *topoi* that provide a grounding for what is familiar and expected of cultural identities (such as depressed persons, millennials, or white people, for instance). Like Olson's study of indigenous cultures, the shared cultural knowledge necessary to make implicative judgements about individuals as part of collectives plays a key role in memetic practice—and memes' ambivalence allows for different kinds of judgments, depending upon the discourses upon which one draws to make sense of the memes' enthymemes.

Memes as topic (i.e., *topos*) are commonplaces that are shared through a digital social body. For Marshall (2001), online space (as locale or *topos*):

> both expresses and reflects the status and reflection of participants and produces a "mood," or mode of being, which can apparently reduce the inherent divergence of meaning, and help the formation of commonalities, which may help the survival of a particular class of individuals in an uncertain world. (p. 95).

That is, the collective thoughts that create the "mood" of respective locales online have persuasive influence over the places they inhabit. However, Marshall writes from an era before the advent of mobile phones (at least, before they were ubiquitous). His argument is even more intriguing now in an era when online interaction takes place in a greater variety of contexts than through a stationary computer, especially given the vague boundaries between "online" and "offline" in all forms of digital communication. Like Yancey's (2019) tombstones, the *topoi* of depression symptoms and meanings proliferate online and off, gaining new and intriguing meanings as they go. The motion of depression memes through various cultural and discursive spaces affords them ambivalent meaning(s) in the spaces they inhabit (digital and otherwise).

Thus, I view memes as *topoi* to understand their ambivalent meanings in internet spaces, particularly as purveyors of what it means to have depression. First, however, I must establish the connection between *topoi* and enthymeme, thus linking them as implicative commonplaces shared online. Memes' implicative, collective, and circulatory tendencies underscore their ambivalence, further illuminating their tendency to establish hard-to-describe topics online (depression, for example).

Therefore, combining enthymeme with topic provides another way to view depression memes ambivalently and thus tease out some of their potential meanings. To some scholars, enthymemes partially operate through the use of common knowledge (Walton, 2001). Scott (2002) explored the ways that:

> enthymemes can be built partly around *topoi*. At the same time, an enthymeme is something different from and more than a *topos*. An enthymeme entails not only a generative structure for an argument but also the argument itself. An enthymeme, in other words, is the actual body of persuasion deployed in a rhetorical context, although some of its premises and proofs may be implicit. (p. 57-58).

In this case, *topoi* (in other words, commonplaces) are especially important, as internet memes are circulated pieces of common knowledge that are shared among social groups. As memes are passed around a social sphere, they become understood as commonalities, since users become familiar with their meanings through repetition. In order to understand a meme, there are *topoi* that the viewer must be aware of (such as the meme's platform, style, tropes, etc.).

Viewed as digital *topoi,* memes "simultaneously provide anonymity and connection" as they travel through online spaces (Said & Silbey, 2018, p. 104). For example, Twitter, to the user, feels "real, unmediated, and unrestrained even as it may be anonymous, distant, and unmoored" (Said & Silbey, 2018, p. 107). The tension between "real" and "not real" held together in one space is significant, as internet users must tease out the differences for themselves. As mentioned previously, Czyzewski (2001) wrote at the turn of the 21st century about the "collective consciousness" of anxiety pervasive in Western society (p. 265). These examples illustrate the power of *topoi* in digital spaces as creators and reflectors of "current social moods" (Czyzewski, 2001, p. 268).

Through a similar mechanism, memes illustrate the culturescapes they inhabit. That is, *topoi* hold power within the collectives in which they operate, and memes are made powerful through a user's ability to be "in the know" online. Viewed this way, memes offer shared internet topics for virtual interaction. Cursed images, as one example, are knowable only to those who have known them previously through circulation. A first encounter is not enough; one must also have experience with related *topoi* in order to understand why and how an image is cursed. Similarly, depression memes ask their viewers to be familiar with a wide variety of discourses and cultural beliefs about memes, depression, personhood, and a variety of other implicative knowledges in order to understand the joke. Put another way, "*topoi* are collective thoughts, some of which are common to many subjects, and some of which pertain to specific subjects" (Marshall, 2001, p. 92).

Linking internet memes to the concept of *topoi* allows us to unpack the social moods they create and reflect. For Czyzewski (2001), "the anxieties of our times" is an important social *topos* that influences our modern understandings. Post-modernity, according to Czyzewski, was to free us from universal tropes, but we have merely replaced them through digital platforms. Similarly, memes are repeatable nodes of shared understanding that allow for the reifying of cultural understandings of depression, which has long been a hotly debated *topos* in Western medical culture. To that end, my sample illustrates that depression memes tend, either explicitly or implicitly, to participate in various *topoi* of depression, sometimes from the perspective of an individual sufferer, sometimes from the perspective of society as a whole, and sometimes a combination of both.

Generally, depression memes use depression symptoms colloquially, rather than medically, although memes sometimes draw on precise descriptions familiar to anyone conversant with the DSM-V (American Psychiatric Association, 2013). Although there are a variety of ways one could interpret depression memes and memetic depression discourses and online, my analysis suggests that the circulatory *topos* of depression online is that of globalized, collective suffering. In the following sections, I analyze examples from my sample and contextualize them within the greater discourse of depression in contemporary society.

The online realm, thus, marks a staged battleground for wider discourses and experiences offline, whose boundaries are shaky at best. Depression memes rely on a widely circulated discourse of mental health that permeates online and offline spaces, moving back and forth at will. Internet users debate, discuss, and relate over symptoms of depression through a wide variety of discursive objects, including memes. The memes in this section rely heavily on discourses of mental health to build the affective jokes discussed in the previous chapter, but with the added element of circulation. That is, these memes rely on the movement of memetic tropes, practices, and formats, which have circulated through various media; viewers must be familiar with memetic discourses to grasp the discursive elements within—and may draw different conclusions about what the memes' humor reveals, even while holding mixed emotions about each. Lastly, the memes in this section utilize motion through discursive spaces and movement through physical space. In these examples, affect is an underlying force built upon by the movement of affective *topoi* of depression symptoms; sharing, as they say, is caring.

Since depression has been difficult to define over the centuries, enthymematic *topoi* in memes have stepped in to describe it for internet users. I have chosen a subset of memes from my sample for analysis here to describe a few topics habitual to depression memes (for the full sample of this memetic category, see Appendix B). These memes, overall, deal with what depression "looks" like (as in Chapter Three) but on a more collective scale. That is, these memes make effable the ineffable experience of depression but do so with an awareness of humans in relation to others (in other words, the Everyone with the emphasis on "every" instead of "one").

Specifically, the topics carried by depression memes fall under the larger *topos* of suffering, sometimes roughly corresponding to depression symptoms but often used more vaguely as indicators of widespread angst. The four *topoi* I highlight here include 1) an emphasis on "the struggle" of daily life, 2) self-hatred, 3) questioned authority/ownership over depression, and 4) an eagerness to die. I use meme examples to represent each of these topics, but more examples can be found in the Appendices (see Appendix B). I use these examples as rough indicators of the overall modes of expression utilized in these memes to highlight their role in the wider discourse of depression and to further build toward depression memes as ambience (which I discuss in the next chapter). As these memes speak to collective suffering, they potentially reach out to, or circulate, among those who do not experience clinical depression but who nonetheless *feel* depressed in other way. These four *topoi* merely illustrate a few ways that depression memes describe suffering in post-modernity; they paint a picture of what it means the be the suffering Everyperson in relation with suffering Others.

Topic One: The Struggle

Depression memes depict daily living as inherently rooted in struggle, although more recent memes use "same" or "mood" as tacit complicity in that same struggle as a grander construct. In other words, depression memes assume an inherent *heaviness* of daily life. By and large, memes about the struggle take for granted an inherent difficulty in daily existence, habitually equating the experience of life with the experience of strife. For instance, Figure 4.2 utilizes a character from a popular meme *topos*: the Nickelodeon television series *Spongebob Squarepants*, which is also often used in depression memes throughout the web, not merely on Reddit. In the meme, the character Plankton falls resignedly into a swirling vortex that the caption designates "a pit of despair and stress;" indeed, he casually sucks on the straw of the drink he holds in his hand as he falls backward into the void (see Figure 4.2). Ambivalently, the meme juxtaposes humor and suffering, but also the discourses of children's television with mental illness, creating humor through the contrast in elements in the meme and its relationship to worldly circumstance.

Figure 4.2

Jus Ain't Fightin It

When life is sucking u into a pit of despair and stress but u really jus ain't fightin it anymore

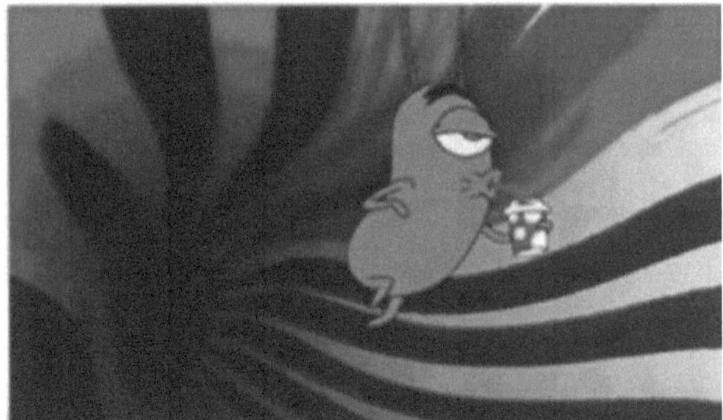

The meme in Figure 4.2 asks significant questions about mental health, the self, and appropriate reactions to life's "despair and stress" (which is taken for granted), all in one image and a caption. To understand Figure 4.2, a viewer must be familiar with the show and the meme format of image+text, but also must be familiar with a nuanced interpretation of "despair and stress" and its relationship to mental wellbeing (or rather, the lack thereof), along with the youth culture that pervades the memescape. Significantly, the meme in Figure 4.2 never mentions depression by name. The meme only refers to the tendency of "life" to bring one "despair and stress," along with the Everyperson's acceptance of these circumstances as a matter of course. This creates an imprecision of meaning when considering one's own experience of depression. Depending on one's insider or outsider status in the discourse, how is one to interpret the meme? Individual experience is not taken into account; instead, the meme implies that "everyone" is part of the depression "club" by assuming that life sucks people down into suffering.

The depiction comes from the shared cultural tropes of television, television characters, memes, and meme formats, but also the shared *topos* of "life," "despair and stress," and the shared knowledge of the vortex. More importantly, the circulation of objects in the meme assists with its meaning, as viewers must be aware of themselves as in-relationship with a variety of cultural, discursive, and memetic tropes to participate. As cited previously, enthymeme not only "plays on an audience's assumptions but can also help shape those assumptions" (Scott, 2002, p. 61). Similarly, the meme draws on audience assumptions about depression, *Spongebob,* memes, and other cultural topics to build the joke. For instance, Plankton's character in the television show starts off as a villain but later becomes a more sympathetic anti-hero, an interesting choice when considering the self as "fightin" depression, as the character could be seen as "mellowing out" over time. Viewers of the show and the meme are better able to appreciate the nuances of the joke when familiar with these circulatory knowledges, although lower levels of knowledge can be helped along as the discourse further "shapes" viewer assumptions.

One the one hand, the assertion that "u" "just ain't fightin it anymore" describes a *topos* of depression as conqueror. On the other hand, another interpretation might emphasize a sarcastic interpretation of depression as something that we purposefully allow to defeat us. There are other interpretations, of course, but a further takeaway from this meme is its embeddedness: in popular culture, in carryout drinks with straws, in "life" as "despair and stress," and the experience of depression in daily living. The enthymematic leaps between these *topoi* emphasizes depression as *in circulation*—the implication is that we are all in the swirling vortex together, so we understand the joke. Like the cursed image at the beginning of this chapter, viewers can know the image depicts depression because the viewer might carry the same cultural "baggage" and can thus relate to the "despair and stress" in the image.

As the meme in Figure 4.2 refers to merely to "life" in general, the meme in Figure 4.3 emphasizes the longevity of the struggle. Mimicking a Wikipedia page (which suggests complexity and depth in chronicling one's life history), the meme refers to the experience of a "first date," wherein the date asks the Everyperson to "tell me about yourself" (see Figure 4.3). The mock-Wikipedia article lists "Early Life," "The First Disaster," "Additional Disasters," and "Public Embarrassment" as headings in the article; the image is cut off, implying that there are more disasters not pictured. As an enthymeme, the image invites the viewer to fill in the details of those disasters by not providing any specifics on what that life might have involved. Although no mention is made of depression or any other mental health diagnosis, the meme ambivalently pokes fun at the coming-of-age experience and the inherent struggle (presumably) found therein. By juxtaposing the seriousness of a Wikipedia page (primarily a website of factual information) with the humor of sarcasm, the meme ambivalently provides mixed emotions regarding dating when depressed. Indeed, the use of Wikipedia is coded "intellectual," perhaps aligning with the tendency of Reddit and Tumblr to riff on the young, edgy, intellectual depressed person as an archetype (as in the popular memetic designation, "me, an intellectual").

Figure 4.3

So Tell Me About Yourself

on a first date

Her: so tell me about yourself

Me:

Contents [hide]

1 Early Life

2 The First Disaster

3 Additional Disasters

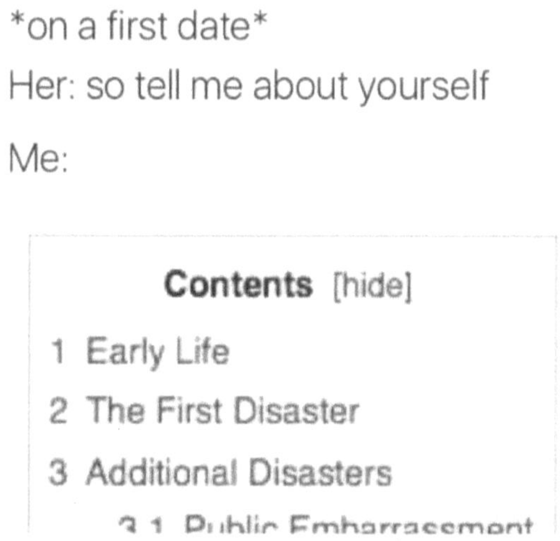

Further, the meme ambivalently connects to a variety of discourses about the appropriateness of disclosure, the navigation of relationships, and other complexities of daily living while depressed. The usage of first date seems significant, as the meme could be described as depicting a "coming out" moment for depression; to talk about oneself as a series of difficulties conflates "self" with "struggle." This meme requires contextual knowledge about dating in certain (primarily Western) cultures, a familiarity with Wikipedia and its format, and a connection to the experience described in the meme. As Prenosil (2012) argued, the premises of the enthymeme are "hidden" within a network of possibilities; similarly, by making enthymematic, circulatory jumps between these (and other) elements, the meme suggests that the transition from "Early Life" to the point of first dates necessitates some disasters in between, then further allows the Everyperson to fill in personal experience. The circulatory enthymeme here is one of "cringey" affect filled in through enthymematic leaps, both through the viewer's/creator's lifespan and the cultural experiences of developing relationships while experiencing the symptoms of depression.

In another example, the meme in Figure 4.4 draws upon the memetic trope, "guess i'll die," to depict the depression symptom of "nauseous because i haven't eaten, can't eat because i'm nauseous" (see Figure 4.4). This meme refers more specifically to a depression symptom (decreased appetite) than many of the examples in the sample, ambivalently joking about a daily practice and the inherent struggles associated with it (in this case, not eating due to nausea). To understand this meme, one must be familiar with the "guess i'll die" meme, which is typically used in highly ambivalent terms. As a form of heavy irony, the meme feigns stoicism about a problem, either large or small, that may or may not require an urgent response. The punchline usually refers to a lack of response to that problem, inverting expectations to create the humor (although the meme usually features a young girl making the same expression as the man in this example, a further layer of irony). The complexity of daily living forms an ambivalent, affective picture of life as rooted in difficulty and yet rendered absurd by the sheer incongruity of it. By mixing the energy of "guess I'll die" memes with depression and the difficulties of keeping oneself alive, the meme creates a multi-layered, ironic jab at the individual experience of suffering in a self-deprecating appeal to the wider world of depression and memes.

Figure 4.4

Guess I'll Die

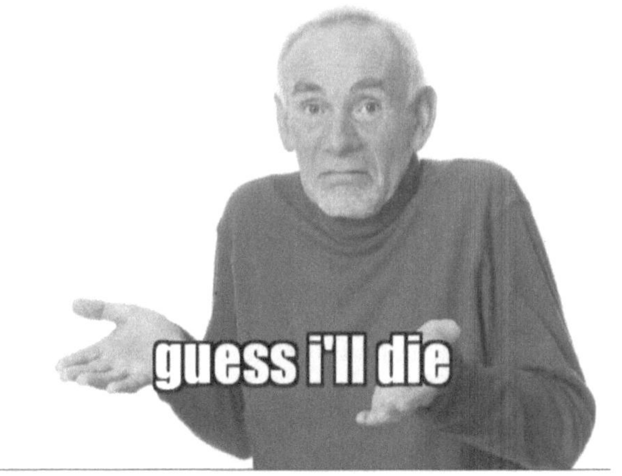

The meme in Figure 4.4 hinges on a person's familiarity with the experience of lack of appetite along with a familiarity with the meme format; the enthymematic leap comes when the viewer connects the two. Prenosil's (2012) "vast, dark reservoir" (p. 298), fits especially well here, as the vast, dark reservoir of knowledge of the individual experience of depression collides with the wider world of memes through circulation in this meme by connecting medical symptoms with the embodied experience of living without appetite. Like many depression memes, Figure 4.4 draws upon a daily "normal" experience that, due to depression, is rendered complex and somehow also funny through its irony. In this case, the ambivalent affects point out the inherent struggle woven into every aspect of daily life with depression and invite the viewer into an in-group of knowing about the experience.

Topic Two: Self-Loathing

The struggle, as a topic, draws upon a variety of circulatory knowledges to describe inherent suffering in the mundane parts of living, which, according to these examples, is a highly ambivalent experience. Similarly, the *topos* of self-loathing draws upon a variety of depression symptoms to depict daily living as a source of hatred for oneself. The memes in the topic of self-hatred draw upon memetic tropes to explore ambivalent narratives of the self as unlovable, often utilizing self-deprecating jokes. For instance, Figure 4.5 sends out a general "life hack" to anyone that needs it; life hacks, in and of themselves, are a memetic practice that offers life advice to anyone who might read it. Life hack memes are part of a vast internet repository of how-to videos, jokes about outdated infomercials, and actual "life hacks," which are brief tips designed to make the reader's life easier (in other words, a short cut allowing a person to be more productive).

Figure 4.5

Life Hack

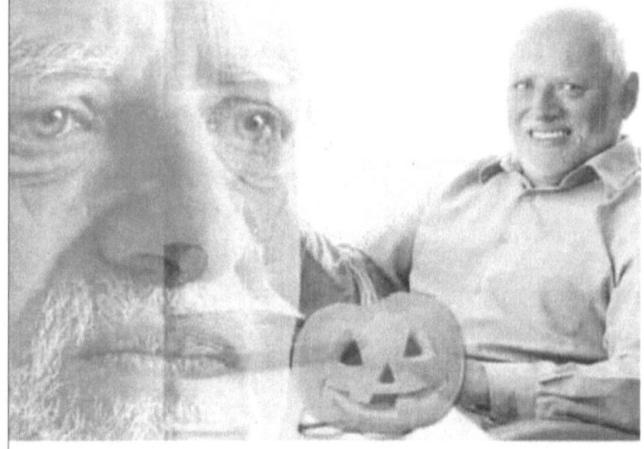

Viewers of this meme require at least a cursory knowledge of these various cultural items to get the joke, along with knowledge of "Hide the Pain Harold," the man featured in the image. Harold has been super-imposed multiple times onto the image, another memetic trope indicating emotion, usually wistful sorrow or confused reverie.

The caption suggests that pumpkin carving is a good activity to "distract you from the fact that you're also a lifeless round object putting on a fake smile" (see Figure 4.5). The use of "lifeless," and "round," are significant: lifeless refers to "dead inside" (as indicated by the reference to being an object and putting on a fake smile) and round refers to a lack of physical fitness. The general "you" in this meme is a subtle implication that everyone must relate to the image—this is not a "depressed person coping tip" but a globalized "life hack." That is, everyone is expected to recognize and benefit from the need to distract themselves from the common human experience of hiding the pain (Figure 4.5). The juxtaposition of the two faces further underlines the ambivalence of feeling expressed in the meme, which emphasizes holding one's feelings in in public spaces.

The circulatory awareness of the "you" (or self) as subject to weight gain, listlessness, and faking a smile points to an awareness of the generalized other as also in distress. The usage of specific depression symptoms in this nonlocal, ambivalent way provides an intriguing critique of personhood; what about "life" requires "hacks" of this kind? The meme poses the question without offering an answer, but enthymematically jumps to the assumptive claim that people in general need the advice regarding these particular problems. Although the meme is ultimately a joke, the circulatory enthymeme(s) contained therein ask complex questions about personhood and suffering by pointing to specific depression symptoms as examples. The implication is that to be a human is to need to "Hide The Pain" like Harold, a circulatory Everyperson in relationship with others. In particular, the Everyperson here struggles with body image, has low self-esteem, and hides their emotions in public spaces (according to the meme), thus indicating a connection to the trope of self-loathing often utilized in depression memes.

Another example of self-loathing in depression memes (see Appendix B) uses text only, captured as an image from Twitter and re-posted on Reddit. The user Tweets, "when u clean ur room so well, that the only trash left is u" (see Appendix B), playing on the idea that the person thinks they are worthless, good only to be thrown away. "Trash" is an internet slang term (in which one must be sufficiently entrenched to get the nuances of it) referring to a human being as worthless and commonly used in depression memes. Cultural enmeshment online invites an attunement to ideas such as these; memes are only one site of usage, and yet an ambivalent joke about "trash" admirably "encapsulates" (Aune, 2003) multiple tropes about depression found online through enthymematic leaps. The mixed feelings of humor, fatigue, bitterness, self-loathing, and a variety of other emotions ambivalently invite the viewer to share in a collective appreciation of suffering by laughing at the memer and themselves as worthless "trash" to be taken out. As a visual enthymeme, the post invites us to fill in the gaps by imagining our own (presumably messy) rooms and the "trash" within: "u."

A final example I draw upon for this topic is found in Figure 4.6, which utilizes a character from the children's animated film *Cars.* The usage of an anthropomorphic racecar and a plastic bag as the Everyperson is interesting here, especially given the objectifying tendencies of the last two meme examples (e.g., "lifeless round object," and "trash") as stand-ins for human beings. Here, it seems, the Everyperson is represented by an inanimate object animated for the purposes of entertainment and glorified for the sake of an ambivalent joke about excessive crying (see Figure 4.6). The affective embodiment of a human being in a plastic bag, coupled with a smiling racecar, provides ambivalent affects but further connects likeminded viewers in a *topos* of the related elements. For instance, in the subtitles included in the image, the character utters a line that represents his tendency toward over-confidence resulting in disaster. Enthymematically, the meme implies that the Everyperson is sarcastically proud of themselves for being the "winner" at something they do not want to do in the first place.

The ambivalent interpretations of the Everyperson in Figure 4.6 exist in a variety of circulatory knowledges about that character, the situation, the experience of "break downs," plastic bags, durability, the environment, and others, including a pun about cars and humans "breaking down" (see Figure 4.6). The variety of nuanced layers combine in a *topos* that hinges on the self as loathsome; by bragging on one's ability to do something undesirable with speed and agility, the meme both praises and criticizes the self in a complex intersection of circulatory tropes. The meme's enmeshment in a variety of discursive knowledges surrounding depression echoes the other examples in this *topos*, which overall depict the self as an object worthy of hatred. By referencing various memetic knowledges, the *topos* of self-loathing assumes a shared hatred of self. Self-loathing, as a topic, assumes the Everyperson is someone deserving of criticism, especially due to ineptitude, lethargy, and other dimensions of worthlessness, often referred to as "trash" (for more examples of this trope, see the appendices). Although the meme never references crying directly, the reference to a "break down" typically involves an emotional outburst after a prolonged period of stoicism, at least as used in depression memes. The character depicted in the image is an ambivalent one, serving both protagonistic and antagonistic roles throughout the film.

Figure 4.6

I Am Speed

When a plastic bag takes 1000 years to break down but you took only one night
I am speed

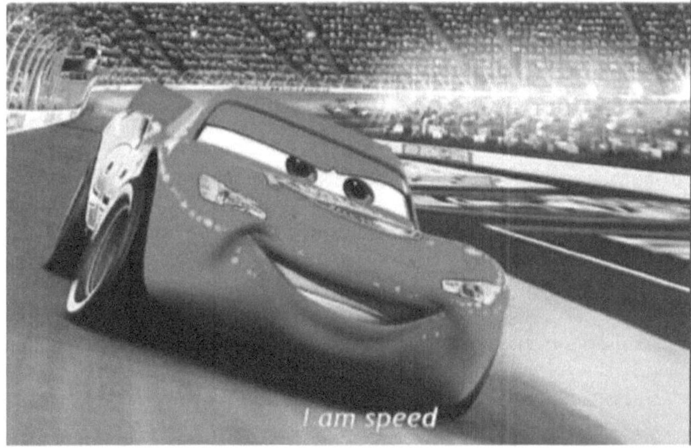

Topic Three: Authority

The memes in the topic of authority ask, essentially: Who owns my depression? Who has the right to define, describe, diagnose, experience, and treat it? By interrogating ownership, these memes discuss complex, ambivalent topics about health, diagnosis, treatment, and other cultural discourses, including a variety of meme discourses and depression itself. As I noted previously, *Spongebob* is a popular meme source, and the show appears again in Figure 4.7, which depicts "How I imagined depressed people as a kid," and "actual depressed people" (Figure 4.7). The two images depict a minor character from *Spongebob.* On the left, which depicts how the meme subject viewed depression when they were "a kid," the character's body movements suggest that of despair: his hands (or rather, fins) are held before his face, the mouth gaping in a dynamic expression of sadness—every limb seems to be in motion with emotion. In the "actual depressed people" box, the same character holds still, wide-eyed and tight-lipped. The right-hand image is also slightly blurry, which could be merely a by-product of quick editing; however, blurriness in meme images is a common practice faintly reminiscent of the "cursed" images from the introduction of this chapter and might (or might not) have been deliberate (although the ambivalence is significant, regardless).

In the space of one meme, the meme-maker chronicles a coming-of-age, critiques a centuries-old discourse, and pokes fun at themselves and everyone else regarding their level of awareness regarding depression. Prenosil's (2012) ontological "relationality among entities" (p. 280) suggests that the act of imagining depressed people and then learning what a depressed person is "actually" like is an enthymematic leap as one "connects the dots" over the course of one's life, so to speak. Further, it hints at both an awareness of self and others that takes vast knowledges of depression into account, especially with an awareness of self in relation to other (especially appropriate in a sub-Reddit for depression memes).

Figure 4.7

Actual Depressed People

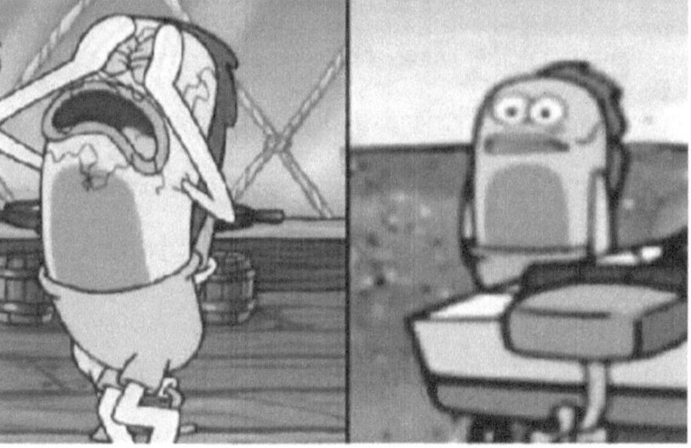

Particularly, the meme implies a familiarity with depression as a circulatory knowledge, perhaps experienced by the meme-maker and perhaps not. The meme marries cultural knowledges of depression in society with pop culture references in a succinct, ambivalent critique of mental health discourses, hinting at a certain "woke" ability to know and understand what depression looks like. The idea of being "woke" (aware, educated, active) about depression through circulatory knowledges is particularly significant; it suggests that the meme image serves as a node of recognition in a discourse of caring about depression as a *topos*.

Viewers are expected to relate to these cultural knowledges (or at least be aware of them) to commune with the joke, further highlighting the embeddedness of the meme. The circulatory nature of the *Spongebob* meme and its depicted relationship to depression illustrates a comfortability with a variety of discourses, between which the meme switches effortlessly. In another example, Figure 4.8 requires a viewer to understand "your mom" (and by extension, "your dad") jokes, the drinks machine meme format, depression, youth culture, and other nuanced knowledges of depression. The meme depicts a hand (labeled "my dad") pressing two buttons to combine two varieties of soft drink in one fast food cup; the left-hand button is labeled "your depression is your fault," and "depression doesn't exist," implying that the assumed Everyperson's father is intolerant and unsupportive.

The circulatory entrenchment of depression and the various elements of the meme underscore the complexities of the discourse as portrayed in memes, as it incorporates a wide variety of these discourses in its purview. As enthymematic leaps are conducted "in [the] mind" (Miller & Bee, 1972, p. 202), a potential mental process of depressed individuals play out visually in this meme; the embodied tension of the hand pressing the drink buttons seems to mirror the mental tension of ownership of depression. By teasing out the ambivalence in the tension, the meme indicates a shared frustration through the humorous release of a "your dad" joke. Typical "your dad" jokes use a stereotypical middle-aged father as the butt of the joke; this one goes further by critiquing the irony of disbelieving in depression while simultaneously insisting that the depression one does not have is one's fault.

Figure 4.8

My Dad

your depression is your fault
depression doesn't exist
Sprite
Coke
PUSH
PUSH
my dad
44oz

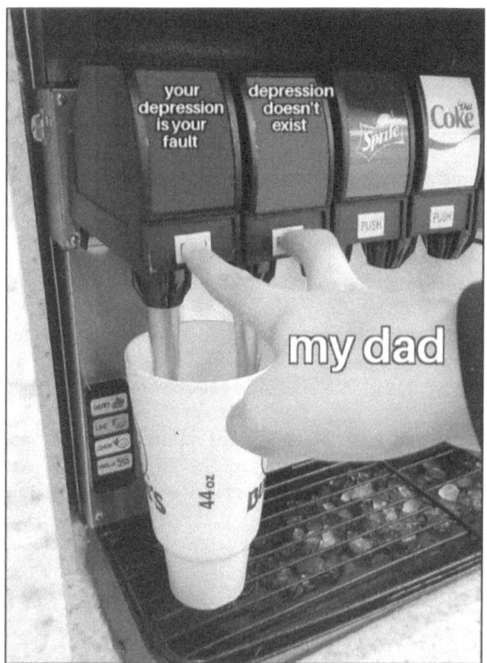

Again, this example critiques a centuries-long discussion of the nature of self and wellbeing, but also incorporates a variety of memetic and social nuances, including the meme format, gender roles, generational rivalries, American soda fountain culture, and the definition of depression, to name a few. The meme exists at the center of a complex circulation of *topoi,* which carry a multiplicity of meanings. Viewers must relate to at least some of the tropes contained therein, which circulate in a multi-layered arena of mental health discourses with facility.

More significantly, the meme makes complex claims about depression discourses, interrogating the contradictory, ambivalent claims that depression can simultaneously be a figment of a sufferer's imagination as well their own fault—in other words, somehow real and not real at the same time. Affectively, the meme holds a variety of conflicting emotions in the enthymematic leaps, suggesting frustration, sorrow, mild humor, bitterness, fondness, and others. However, the meme further calls these affects into being through suggestion of shared *experience,* implying that anyone who views the meme must also carry background knowledge of this kind. The cultural "baggage" of parental disconnect provides a peer-level connection, as (presumed) children of (presumed) non-depressed fathers bond over the affective experience. Again, the implication is that the Everyperson is well aware of the nuanced discourses of depression; further, they must defend themselves against an onslaught of misinformation regarding the existence of depression and who has the right to make claims about it.

As Poe's Law states (Phillips & Milner, 2017), it is impossible to tell the difference between seriousness and irony online; depression memes like this one, in particular, highlight the mixed feelings inherent in the discourse through the tensioned struggle depicted in the various elements of the meme. Although every meme in the discourse is arguably both "funny" and "not funny" at the same time, this particular example illustrates that depression memes have a peculiar ability to be just as uncomfortable as comfortable, which is especially prevalent in Reddit memes (although takes place in depression memes throughout the web). Indeed, this meme has almost no comic "release," but maintains the tension from top to bottom, emphasizing the difficulties of subjective experience when depressed. In terms of *topos*, the meme draws upon a variety of circulatory discourses but emphasizes the internal struggle within that discourse. The enthymematic leap hinges on those discursive elements in a way that invites others into the "club" of suffering from being misunderstood.

Similarly, Figure 4.9 utilizes the popular meme topic of therapy, or rather, the therapist as a character in a widespread memetic trend. The therapist, as a cultural trope, has begun to play a significant role in a variety of memes beyond the bounds of self-avowed mental health memes, as in this example (which does not mention a particular diagnosis). In the caption, the therapist informs the patient that they can "be anything you want to be," to which the invisible subject promptly responds with an image of a young man lying face down on a highway, near a sign that says, "speed bump" (see Figure 4.9). The combination of a therapist joke with the speed bump image invites the viewer into an interpretation of depression steeped in a circulation of discourses surrounding therapy, therapists, suicide, and youth culture. Enthymematically, the meme draws upon therapy as a construct and suicide as a popular joke trend, requiring the viewer to be familiar with at least these memes to get the joke. Admittedly, this meme could easily fit in the next topic ("Eager To Die") but fits here more succinctly due to its emphasis on the therapist as a subject.

The ambivalence of joking about therapists opens a circular interrogation, suggesting that therapists are simultaneously both "right" and "wrong." The localized experience of depression contrasted with the globalized process of diagnosis and treatment plays out in memes of this type as a circulatory trope. Therapists memes, in general, depict the therapist as helpful, friendly, and supportive, bordering on naïve, while the patient is portrayed as cynical, knowledgeable, and often superior through skepticism (as evidenced in several examples throughout this book). Therapist meme images usually depict the patient as a sarcastic, witty, and winning figure who knows much more than the therapist about what it means to be mentally ill.

Although therapist memes are popular on many social media platforms, the sample from the sub-Reddit only contained a few examples, perhaps due to a tendency to rather over-emphasize suicide memes in the edginess of "dark" Reddit (although this meme incorporates both the therapist and suicide as a meme). Tumblr is more commonly known for therapist memes, although therapist memes, as "safer" than other forms of depression meme, often find their way onto other platforms (such as Facebook, which houses some depression memes but is not known colloquially for doing so). The therapist as a rhetorical figure enjoys a sort of parental, yet mistaken, authority role on many platforms, as therapy itself is de-stigmatized in various places around the web.

Still, this interpretation is laced with nuance, as attending to the irony and sarcasm in these memes provides alternative interpretations of the therapist as ultimately more informed about the "right" ways to "do" mental illness. No matter which interpretation(s) one chooses, the circulatory *topos* of therapists, therapy, mental illness, memetic practices, and other cultural knowledges come into play in memes such as these. The enthymematic leap comes in as users navigate the various depictions of therapists, therapy, diagnosis, and treatment; the viewer's own experience steps in to fill in the gaps.

Figure 4.9

Anything You Want To Be

Therapist: You can be anything you want to be
Me:
SPEED
BUMP

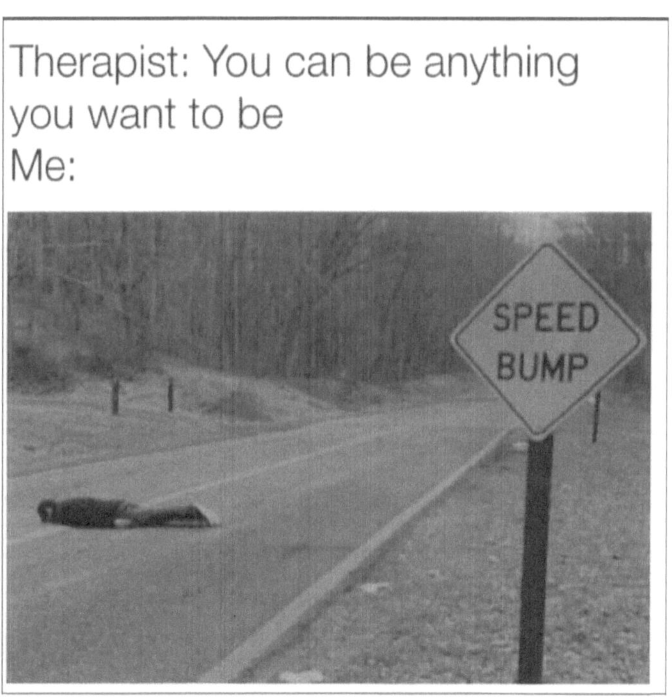

Like the cursed image at the beginning of this chapter, the "curse" of treatment as a baggage colors viewer interpretation, like the "the binding forces of shared information circulating in an organic system" which, Carey (2009, p. 7) argued, make society possible. The implication is that people in therapy are "in the know" and the therapist is not, for how can anyone (even a trained professional) truly know what it is like to be the depressed person? The answer is ambivalent, since joking about being a speed bump is humor of the absurd; and yet, the questions remain as therapy memes, as a *topos*, circulate through the depression meme community and the wider internet as a whole. This permeability becomes especially important in the next chapter; for now, it is enough to make note of the ability of circulatory rhetoric to "rearrange collective life" (Gries, 2013, p. 336).

Topic Four: Eager to Die

The last topic I highlight in this chapter reflects a fondness for death, dying, and joking about dying (often by suicide, though not always). For instance, Figure 4.10 draws upon a popular meme format, the Drake Hotline Bling meme, also known as Drakeposting. This is a popular meme format using screenshots from a music video, where memers use a common template of Drake in the "Don't Like/Like" format (see Figure 4.10). The Drake format for depression memes is popular enough that my sample contained multiple examples (in fact, see Appendix B for another similar to this one). Although the Drake meme has been used in multiple ways, I use this example due to the succinct depiction of a wider attitude toward suicide in depression memes. This example depicts Drake shunning "actual jokes" in favor of "suicide memes," indicating that suicide memes are much better than "actual" jokes (a label left entirely open to the viewer's interpretation).

Figure 4.10

Actual Jokes

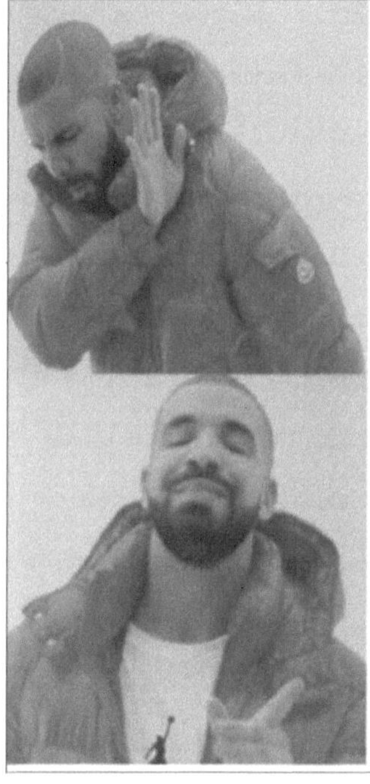

Joking that suicide memes are the superior form of joke is a clever meta-joke, of course; however, it also serves the dual purpose of questioning the value of jokes and suicide memes as forms of humor. Without mentioning depression, Figure 4.10 explores the utility of suicide memes in mental health discourse; memes, as the internet suggests, are the "cure" for depression, and yet here are also implied to be the cause. More broadly, though, Figure 4.10 draws on cultural tropes to make claims about the cultural value of jokes and suicide memes, as well as suicide as a value-laden topic within that culture. As Akram et al (2020) noted, depression memes tended to be funnier to those experiencing the physical symptoms of depression. By inverting the expectation of suicide as undesirable, the meme plays with aspects of cultural normativity by creating an in-group of those who find the joke humorous (similar to the cursed image's ability to create in-groups through exclusion of outgroups through discomfort). Circulatory beliefs about life, death, humor, and sorrow are flipped upside down in the meme, suggesting alternative ways to view mental health and illness when one is "in the know."

The implicative leaps in the meme in Figure 4.10 suggest a collective appreciation of suicide memes, as well as a collective knowledge of what "actual" jokes are. The meme implies that "we" all "know" what a *real* joke is, and still "we" choose to view suicide memes for their ambivalent (and seemingly inherent) value. Although "we" might refer specifically to Reddit users, these *topoi* are found throughout the web. Certainly, a dark meme like this one is "safer" in a platform like Reddit, but the sentiment in the meme refers imprecisely to "we" reminiscent of depression memes across multiple platforms. The viewer is simultaneously invited to poke fun at and enjoy suicide memes as simultaneously worthwhile and worthless.

Drake, in this particular example, is both the Everyperson and Drake himself; by choosing to distance oneself or relate oneself to Drake as a figure, perhaps simultaneously, "we" are invited to appreciate suicide memes as objects of horror and fascination. The meme seems to faintly emanate bitterness; like the cursed image, we are invited to share in mixed emotions with everyone else who gets the joke. One interpretation, of course, is that suicide jokes (and therefore, depression) are "cool;" another interpretation is that only stupid people like Drake would think so (depending on one's opinion of Drake). The ambivalence further underscores the irony in the meme while simultaneously critiquing mental health discourses; perhaps the implication is that "offline" people (or people "IRL") do not understand depression, while online people (or memers) do.

In another popular example, two meme formats merge in a joke about how eager people might be to die (see Figure 4.11). The "Will you press the button?" meme is a common one; it provides two alternatives and a bright red button that the viewer is invited to consider. Similar to the game "would you rather?" (itself a cultural memetic), the button provides a choice and a consequence. For instance, Figure 4.11 suggests that if you push the button, "you will die a painless and peaceful death" but "nobody will miss you and care about your death." In the original meme format, these two ideas are presented as opposites, suggesting that a person must sacrifice the second option for the benefit of the first option. This version, though, is combined with the Spiderman version of this meme, who, in memes, usually makes "bad" decisions deliberately and with enthusiasm; his posture displays triumph as he presses the button as fast as he can. This meme indicates that to die and not be missed would be a mercy, as it indicates a suicide wherein there are no consequences.

Figure 4.11

Will You Press THE BUTTON?

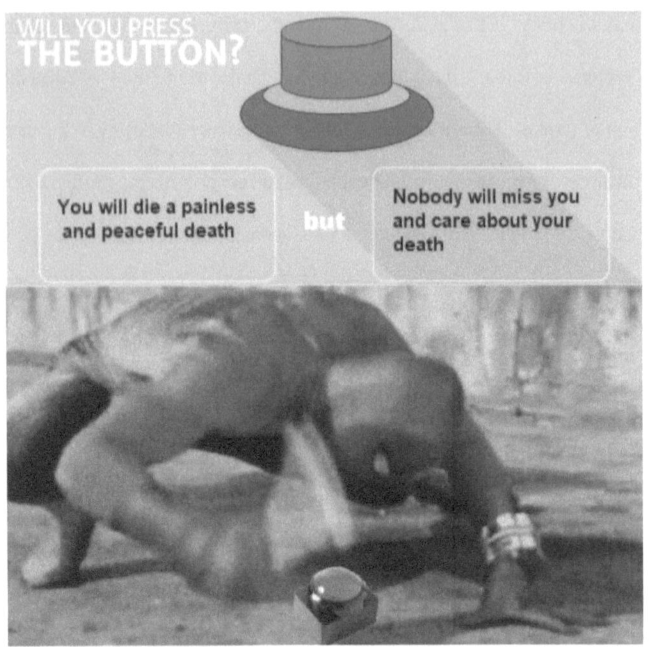

Incidentally, a reverse-image Google search of this particular image reveals dozens of memes in the same format, many using death as the punchline; a few such examples label the Spiderman in the bottom panel "Reddit," suggesting that Reddit is full of people who want to die (Reddit and Tumblr are both internet famous for being a stronghold of depressed bloggers). This self-deprecating, self-aware frankness about suffering is common in depression memes, but especially memes of this flavor, and the more familiar you are with the suffering of Spiderman (and superheroes in general), the more salient the joke. By seeing the Everyperson (with the emphasis placed firmly on *every*) as Spiderman, viewers can share in a collective fictionalization that admits the possibility of consequence-free suicide. The reference to suicide without consequences is suggestive, as it seems to indicate depression but not serious depression; Spiderman here stands in for the viewer who wants to die but not enough to hurt anyone by doing it. The popular meme format and its reference to "you" as the subject suggests a widespread desire to end one's life peacefully, painlessly, and without hurting anyone else.

Although the meme in Figure 4.11 is perhaps merely a joke about how foolish Spiderman is, the ambiguity suggests a multi-layered approach. Still, the suggestion that to relate to this joke means a comfortability with suicide is an interesting one, given the stigma surrounding suicide in contemporary Western culture. Suicide memes (such as the ones in this section) are almost pro-suicide activism; although they do not openly support suicide (per se), they offer a playful, subversive platform in which to discuss suicide without provoking any "real" alarm. After all, a meme is just a joke, right? Indeed, this meme illustrates the way internet rhetoric "collapses and complicates" binary structures (Phillips & Milner, 2017) through ambivalence. In the binary question of whether a viewer will choose to press the button or not, the meme upturns the binary by suggesting that there are actually more than two sides to the question. By questioning the validity of traditional understandings of suicide, the Spiderman meme in Figure 4.11 offers a playful, fictional world (that of superheroes and science fiction) in which to explore death as a topic through a joke.

Figure 4.12

Who Is The Most Stupid Here?

WHO IS THE MOST STUPID HERE?
1
2
3
4
Everyone thinks 4 is stupid but honestly 4 is mood

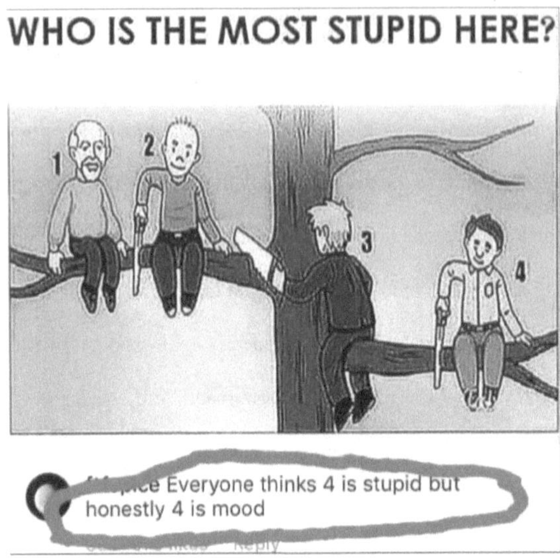

Similarly, the example in Figure 4.12 builds on the idea of casual suicide jokes by suggesting that the fourth person in the image (labeled number 4) is "mood," as indicated by the caption. In other words, the viewer and others are expected to relate to the desire to saw off a branch while sitting on it. The image was already a meme, but the caption (captured with the image) makes it a depression meme. The caption explicitly invokes the "Everyone" ambivalently, by both implying that "Everyone" got the answer wrong, but simultaneously inviting "Everyone" to partake in the "mood" of the man cutting the very branch he is sitting on. As a joke, the viewer is expected to laugh at the assumption that everyone shares the secret desire to die, and yet the meme ambivalently invites the viewer to indulge in the possibility (although others not as entrenched in the discourse might find themselves un-amused or even shocked). The layers point to a suicide joke, a reference to the self as "trash" (stupid and not worth saving), and an eagerness to die all in one meme.

Depression memes in this chapter represent circulatory discourses of the Everyperson as struggling, more or less aligned with depression symptoms. The imprecision of description, ambivalent, complex layering of symptoms, and enmeshment with personhood represent the depressed Everyperson as in relationship with depressed others, part of a globalized "club" of suffering. Since depression memes depict what it means to be a depressed person, they reflect, to some extent, on the humanness of depression. However, memes in this chapter take this line even further by emphasizing the depression within humanity; that is, rather than merely describing *depressed people*, they describe *people*. The effect (or, more accurately, affect) is a depiction of people as depressed. In essence, some of these memes explained what it means to be a depressed person, while some of them described what it means to be a *person*. To be a person is to have depression, as demonstrated by the memes in this chapter (and the additional memes relegated to Appendix B for the practicality of space). Although depression memes supposedly describe the individual experience of diagnosed suffering of depression symptoms, these memes have a tendency to do so imprecisely and without acknowledging the biological factors of depression. Instead, they tend to emphasize the social dimensions of depression by referring to a vague wish to die, generalized inner turmoil, and eagerness for solidarity with others (diagnosed or otherwise).

That is, if the memes in the previous chapter depict what it means to be a depressed person, the memes in this chapter depict what it is to be a depressed person in relation to other depressed persons. Even as these memes describe depression symptoms, they imply degrees of universality of these symptoms, drawing on collectivity and unity through memetic tropes (e.g., pop culture references, meme figures, and other examples). Indeed, depression memes describe depression symptoms beyond a normative discourse of depression, although admittedly they do so on a Reddit designed for depression memes. Instead, these memes enthymemetically and affectively assume widespread awareness of depression, a certain "wokeness" to the traits of the disorder. The in-between premises hint almost at an eagerness to join in the depression "club," or, at the very least, to be seen as knowing about depression's intricacies and vicissitudes. Although this tendency might serve to reduce stigma by educating those in the fringes of the in-group and welcoming them into the middle, it might also gloss over individual experience by assuming that "everyone" understands the nuances of everyday lived experience with depression.

Other memes in this sub-category (see Appendix B), similarly, draw upon memetic and discursive knowledges to interrogate what it means to have depression through a visual exploration of *topoi* of depression. Thus, depression memes as discourse participate in and build upon the discourse of depression, both online and off. The circulatory impetus of moving *topoi* inform and re-inform practices and knowledges of mental health through their usage of a variety of circulatory tropes. Lest that sentence remain circular, let me explain: the circulatory tropes used in memes re-circulate those same and additional tropes, building upon each other into a discursive realm of interconnected knowledge about depression. As these knowledges entangle, disentangle, separate and re-connect, they also participate in an even more deep-seeded discourse: that of the very nature of personhood.

The complex entanglements between humor, self-deprecation, depression, mental health literacy, and an endless variety of other related cultural discourses plays out in memetic practice online. As I have explored throughout this book, depression is trending. More particularly, the nuanced and ambivalent way that memes discuss depression indicates a culture that is deeply familiar with the experience of depression, and comfortable discussing it in public spaces (albeit sometimes in a joking manner). The television characters, public figures, pop culture references, meme formats, depression symptoms, cultural beliefs, and discursive knowledges move through online and offline spaces with ease, swirling together and apart in a many-sided system of information and emotion. As they move, they carry bits of depression with them; to see them is to participate in a grander discourse about what it means to be well and unwell, sane and insane.

Significantly, the memes in this chapter not only draw upon the movement of cultural tropes, pop culture references, depression as discursive *topos,* and other circulatory elements through online spaces, but also the concept of movement itself. Every meme I chose for this chapter (for further examples, see Appendix B) further utilizes motion itself, even in the still images used in the meme. Figure 4.2 suggests movement as a cartoon character falls into a swirling vortex; Figure 4.3 contrasts movement with stillness as the eye moves from one panel to the next. Every single figure in this section and related appendix utilizes motion as part of the meme, in fact. Even Figure 4.10, which depicts a man posing as a speed bump, contrasts the motion of oncoming cars with the deliberate non-motion of lying in the road. The *motion*, or, as the case may be, *non-motion*, of a suffering person adds a layer of nuance to an already nuanced discourse.

Conclusion

Although the circulatory nature of the tropes within each meme and the movement of the meme itself is significant, even more interesting is the usage of *motion* in the memes themselves. This usage of motion underscores the ever-shifting, ever-present undercurrent of depression pervading our society, as evidenced by the casual, ubiquitous jokes made about depression online. Put another way, these memes interrogate the normalcy of depression as experience through the playful exploration of what it means to be a human being. Of course, the presence of these memes on a sub-Reddit about depression memes arguably suggests that the intended audience is depressed people, and so, therefore, these memes merely refer to the experience of diagnosed clinical depression, rather than the united human experience of suffering. However, depression memes do not merely confine themselves to Reddit, nor do their cultural knowledges originate there. Rather, the widespread use of these formats, practices, and tropes indicates a circulatory familiarity with depression, bordering on normalization. In the next chapter, I further explore the memeworld as an indicator and furtherer of the lifeworld through a discussion of memes as ambient rhetoric.

Chapter 5: Attunement

In 2012, Facebook manipulated the positivity and negativity of certain posts for a week as part of a controversial academic study (Hill, 2014). Scholars have criticized the ethics of the study, which was done without users' knowledge or consent (other than the initial agreements users click to accept when joining the site)—an ethically dubious undertaking (Flick, 2016; Hill, 2014; Sellinger & Hartzog, 2016). The study found that users who viewed more negative posts in that week viewed the world as more negative; the positively valanced posts influenced the users positively. Although highly criticized, Facebook's controversial experiment stands as a lesson in *attunement* (Rickert, 2013); that is, Facebook attuned its users to positivity through positive posts and negativity through negative posts. In this chapter I revisit Rickert's (2013) ambient rhetoric, which he describes as "rhetorical attunement" (as described in Chapters One and Two). Then, using examples from my Reddit sample and from the internet at large, I describe depression memes as aspects of our post-modern attunement to suffering.

By becoming more "awake" to positivity or negativity in their social networks, the Facebook users in the controversial study became more attuned to their respective valances; the result was an enlargement of that valance in their perceptions of the world. Although CMC research has looked at emotional contagion online (e.g., Fowler & Christakis, 2008; Hancock, Gee, Ciaccio, & Lin, 2008) and affect theory (as discussed in Chapter Three) discusses contagion of emotion more broadly, attunement is broad-based, nuanced way to view rhetoric as movement and meaning. Memes, I suggest, offer one example of a new media rhetoric that lends attunement to their viewership. Depression memes, in particular, carry knowledges about depression as they move through the affective circulations they inhabit. By demonstrating that ambient interactions with positive posts influenced users to feel more positive and ambient interactions with negative posts influenced users to feel more negative, Facebook's controversial study demonstrated the persuasive influence of "deep" rhetoric, or rhetoric so engrained in the environmental fabrics of reality that rhetors fail to interrogate its power.

I argue, overall, that depression memes represent and re-affirm particular kinds of attunement to suffering, which magnifies and highlights suffering's rhetorical virility in the world(s) it scaffolds. As ethereal materiality, suffering permeates the scaffolding of these worlds via memes, perhaps boosting its sway over human entities in both the human and non-human milieu. Internet memes represent *hisa* (chaos) and *zhama* (blockage) through their formation of elements-in-collision which nevertheless burst forth in explosions of affective release; combined, depression memes are particles of depression symptoms in a zeitgeist of generalized suffering. Lastly, I demonstrate that memes represent creative expressions that partially fulfill Cvetkovich's (2012) assertion of creativity as a potential release for depression conceptualized as social mood.

Ambience

This chapter utilizes ambient rhetoric as concert with affect and circulation. More specifically, ambience is an overarching structure that encompasses affect and circulation within its bounds. Ambience, which signifies a rhetorical dwelling place, does not mean "worldview," which invokes a Western empirical interpretation of viewpoint, suggesting an objective truth "out there" to be discovered (Rickert, 2013). Rather, rhetorical dwelling refers to the position of a total enmeshment that forms the "carpentry" of the world (Rickert, 2013). Ambience recalls McLuhan's (1968) injunction about fish, who know "exactly nothing" about water because they cannot sense the medium they spend their whole lives in. McLuhan's fish-in-water metaphor predates Rickert's ambience by decades, but both capture the sheer inability of rhetors to get out of the media in which they swim.

Ambience, in other words, represents a dwelling out of which we cannot conceive ourselves; we cannot understand anything outside of the water because our entire existence is bound within it. Perhaps the scientific community, Facebook users, and the public at large found the Facebook positivity study so unsettling because, for the first time, they were forced to notice the water. Attunement has consequences, and unconscious attunement is much more comfortable for rhetors who have learned to breathe in particular flavors of air. Attunement reveals and perpetuates ambivalent discourses of unhappiness that both critique and perpetuate a discourse of depression as a public feeling. That is, depression memes seem to say, "I have depression, you have depression, and we all have depression, but where does the responsibility lie?" An ambivalent reading of the internet renders Facebook's experiment with a binary of positivity and negativity is overly simplistic; and yet, the implications of the study are suggestive.

By attuning its users to positivity or negativity without their knowledge or consent, the Facebook company demonstrated the power of unconscious ambience in our daily lives. In my own social media usage, depression memes pop up on a daily basis across all platforms I inhabit. My notice of them mingles with my own attunement(s) to the world at large, coloring my sense of how it operates. Like the positivity/negativity study, my own "water" is flavored by the particles within it. The Facebook users in the experiment, then, can be compared to "fish" who swim in water of varying degrees of positivity and negativity and then are suddenly informed that the valence of their river current had been tampered with.

However, the comparison only goes so far. For one thing, Facebook is only one "pool" of water, and rhetors swim in thousands of pools at any given time. For another, binaries of "positive" and "negative" are much more complex; even the definition of what counts as "positive" and "negative" is ambivalent. Phillips and Milner (2017) suggested that "ambivalence collapses and complicates binaries within a given tradition. Not just between normal and abnormal, but … between then and now, online and offline, and constitutive and destructive" (Phillips & Milner, 2017, p. 13). The collapse of binaries is evident in rhetorics of depression, the experience of which is complex, variable, and largely indefinable (as the examples in Chapter Three demonstrated), and deeply embedded in the circulatory discourses online (as is evidenced in Chapter Four). The positivity/negativity binary breaks down quickly when considering a mental, emotional, and physical condition like depression.

Ambience, coupled with ambivalence, provides a view of depression as both inside of us and outside of us, sometimes carried back and forth via memes. "To inhabit a place," Rickert (2013) argued, "means something different if the human body is less stably bounded than we are accustomed to thinking it to be," and further, "bodies and brains are . . . more plastic and extended than they formerly had been, and we should do the same with our environments; they inhabit us just as we inhabit them" (p. 42). The memes that move through online spaces and in and out of human bodies, similarly, represent a permeability of depressive affects as they move through online and offline spaces. So, as I argued in Chapter Three, depression memes are modes of transport for affective rhetoric, expressed in the elements of the memes themselves. These affects move internally and externally through the human form, taking part in our dwelling within the world.

Throughout this book, I have written about affect theory and circulation theory as building blocks of ambience; now, I bring them together as a more holistic theoretical lens. First, the affective piece of the theory emphasizes that ambience is within and without us, as the boundaries between rhetoric and the self are rendered permeable by the tendency of rhetoric to fill and surround and bind us. Although depression is not Rickert's focus, he comments on its status as an *external* dwelling-place that invites an *internal* attunement to suffering:

> depression as a mood conspicuously transforms how the world shows up for us; the listlessness common to depression is not just the experience of an already preexisting subject; rather, it transforms a person's world so that the world comes to take part in the depression. Depression generates a cut—sundering afflicted persons from their ties to the world and other people, generating further separation that in turn exacerbates the depression. Depression, that is, is mood as attunement in that it permeates the entire situation, not simply the interior mental

> state of the person, which is one reason that overcoming it requires more than an act of will. (Rickert, 2012, p. 146)

Depression as "cut" or severance between the world and others is especially significant, given the communicative attempts of memes to fill in rhetorical gaps between human and non-human agents.

More particularly, "the mind . . . is seen as something implicated in and dispersed throughout complex social and technological systems" in the ambient lifeworld we now inhabit (Rickert, 2013, p. 41). Through technologies, we are literally scattered into the atmosphere of rhetoric; memes are only one way in which we disperse ourselves into the rhetorical ether. No matter how much meme usage a person engages in, they are in many ways dispersed within technological meme systems online, even as meme systems are dispersed within them. A clear example can be found in meme subjects, who often go accidentally viral; without intending to, their faces and identities are literally dispersed throughout the web in fragmentary and complicated ways.

For instance, Laina Morris, who uploaded a video of herself for a contest submission and subsequently went viral, noted that she started seeing her face everywhere and began to feel separate from her identity, resulting in a deep depression as she struggled to re-frame her sense of self (BuzzfeedVideo, 2020). Morris is one of many, but a person does not need to go viral to scatter themselves liberally over many technological platforms; this dispersal of self has consequences that human beings are only now beginning to wrestle with. The "IRL" and "url" blend with each other, requiring a re-framing of our definitions of what it means to be human and non-human.

In a parallel example, memes and memetic practices also permeate the lifeworld, allowing that same dispersal to work in many ways. T-shirts, posters, artwork, tattoos, mugs, clothing accessories, and other material objects carry slogans such as, "wake up, sleep, survive" (Depression Mugs, 2020) or "girls just wanna have serotonin" (Depression Meme, 2020), carrying the *topos* of depression across locales. A t-shirt design from Look Human in the "depression humor" category (tagged and labeled as such on the site) sports a "My life is a Cat-astrophe" (see Figure 5.1) slogan with an image of a crying cat smiling through its tears (Depression Humor, 2020). The affective elements on the t-shirt, which depicts a cat both smiling and crying, further underscores the ambivalence of the discourse (see Figure 5.1). The conflation of "life" with "catastrophe" in the design is especially suggestive alongside several of the memes in my sample, which tend to place the emphasis on life (a relatively external attribution) rather than on disease (a much more internal attribution). The very existence of a "depression" category on a website for trendy shirt slogans is another testament to the power of depression as a cultural force on the internet.

Similarly, a Google search for "depression memes" results in some 188,000,000 hits, including a number of compilation articles, such as "40 memes that might make you laugh if you have crushing depression" (Virzi, 2019), "Seasonal Depression Comes And Goes, But Depression Memes Are Always Around (39 Memes)" (RuinMyWeek, 2020), and "61 Depression Memes That Prove Laughter Is the Best Medicine" (WinkGo, 2020). Countless Facebook pages, Instagram accounts, Tumblrs, Pinterest boards, blogs, imgurs, and Twitter handles are dedicated to depression generally and depression memes specifically, along with countless other platforms; of course, the sub-Reddits in my sample are no exception. Nor is the trend confined to tangible rhetoric or online spaces; "the struggle," "same," "mood," "sad," "big sad," and other memetic slang terms permeate everyday speech, as evidenced by my interactions with memers during classroom instruction and in social gatherings. I have unironically used "the struggle bus" in full sentences for years.

Figure 5.1

My life is a Cat-astrophe

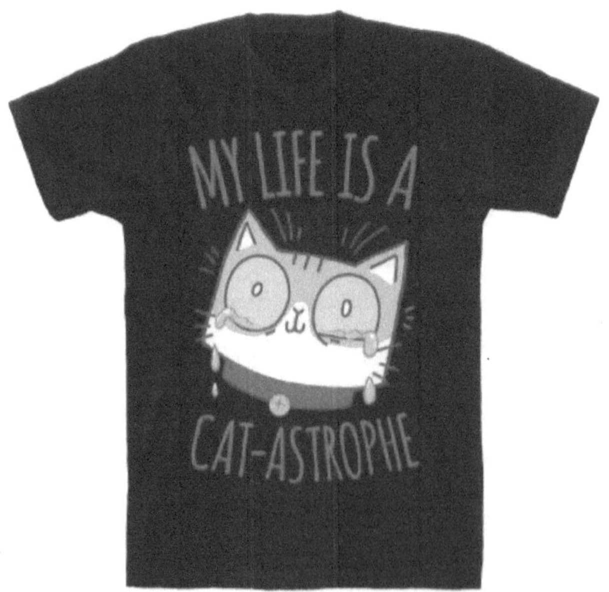

The "my life is a cat-astrophe" (see Figure 5.1) shirt is about depression (or at least, is labeled and grouped with depression shirts online), but makes no explicit reference to diagnosed depression symptoms. Instead of referencing mood swings, sadness, or any other typical depression symptom, it references "life"—a general un-wellness not tied to diagnosis. Similarly, the memes I draw upon in this chapter illustrate a shared attunement toward suffering, partly through depression symptoms and partly through a generalized human condition of "the struggle." By interrogating the ownership and responsibility of depression, depression memes participate in, critique, and perpetuate a generalized depiction of suffering that is sometimes portrayed symptomatically, sometimes more generally, and often both. That is, the ambiguous renderings of depression symptoms point to a complex, sociological #mood of angst that permeates post-modernity not necessarily tied to diagnosis. Instead, depression memes point to a deeper #mood (a generally downcast one).

Attunement to Suffering

As in the previous two chapters, memes in this chapter make enthymematic, affective leaps to make their claims. However, when considering memes as ambient rhetoric, the rhetorical jump being made is one of attunement—it assumes that its audience is attuned similarly. To begin with, depression memes display an awareness of an audience that is (also) depressed, further underscoring the enthymematic, circulatory lifeworld of suffering in which memes operate. In the meme examples in this chapter, internet users seem attuned to suffering as a common human experience, a global #mood.

Further, they seem to understand it as clinical depression even while drawing on symptoms of clinical depression as a widespread characterization for suffering.

In the introduction to this book, I anecdotally referred to a time when I asked myself, "is everyone depressed?" after viewing a quantity of memes that seemed to suggest so. Although that question is, of course, much too rudimentary to be of any practical or theoretical use, my explorations of ambience and depression memes suggest a certain zeitgeist of suffering, roughly corresponding to clinical depression but also more broadly deploring the struggles of contemporary life in parallel to Ahmed's (2010) false promise of post-modern happiness. The falseness of happiness in modernity runs parallel to the ambient "scaffolding" (Rickert, 2013) of depression memes, which represent air molecules in a wider rhetorical atmosphere. Depression memes underline a tendency toward a negative valance, roughly corresponding to the "negative" posts in the Facebook study I cited early in this chapter, although I again emphasize the ambivalence of the discourse. Though still ambivalent, depression memes' tendency to glorify suffering through enthymematic assumptions of generalized misery online.

For example, the meme in Figure 5.2 is an example of a meme that seamlessly interweaves depression symptoms with everyday life. In the examples in this chapter, depression memes loosely correlate depression symptoms with generalized suffering. Moreover, these memes represent suffering as the natural consequence of human existence. As rhetorical particles in a wider rhetorical atmosphere, one cannot easily fathom oneself outside the boundaries of that atmosphere. Suffering, it seems, is woven into the fabric of reality. In his definitive work on ambient rhetoric, Rickert (2013) outlines the ways that rhetoric attunes audiences to particular ways of knowing and being. As with the previous two chapters, the memes in my sample serve as evidence of an ambient dwelling-place that I have become attuned to in my own experiential journey. Throughout this chapter, I use examples from my sample, elsewhere on the internet, and from my own experience to demonstrate how affect, circulation, and ambience illustrate depression memes as threads in a globalized rhetorical tapestry of suffering.

Figure 5.2

Finding The Will To Live

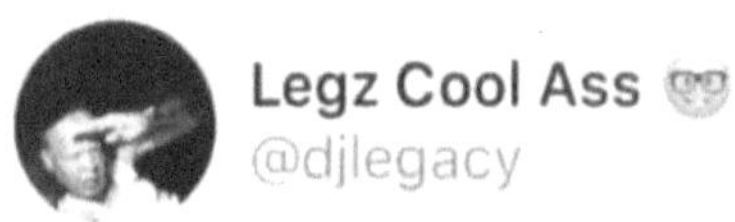

what part of your morning routine takes the longest?

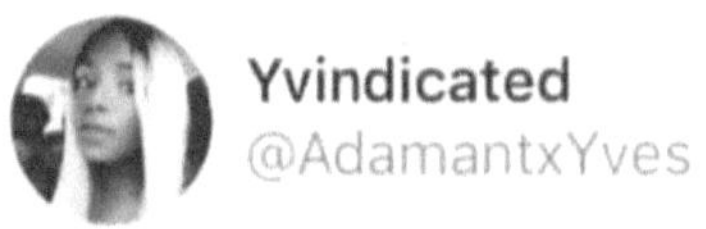

Finding the will to live.

Memes, then, are one example of ambient rhetoric that supports an overall attunement to suffering. While Rickert (2013) focuses on a variety of rhetorical texts, he emphasizes the important ways that new media is "permeating the carpentry of the world" (p. 1) and the material consequences thereof. Rickert (2013) further suggests "that rhetoric circulates through both human and nonhuman elements" of digital media, arguing that digital media are "far-reaching technological extensions of humankind's cognitive processes" (p. 3). Rhetoric exists in an ever-shifting, ambivalent universe, in which "participants create, circulate, and transform shared texts, adding unique and ever-evolving contributions to vast cultural tapestries" (Phillips & Milner, 2017, p. 31). The worldly rhetoricity of attunement takes place in a galaxy of rhetoric including human and non-human actors, which, for the purposes of my study, is a vortex of memes and memers.

For instance, the meme in Figure 5.3 makes a depression joke by blithely suggesting that only depressed people can upvote it. Inviting other depressed people to share in the memeworld in this way suggests an attunement to mutual suffering as shared through meme practices, a self-awareness of a globalized group of memers that post together. The ambivalence in Figure 5.3 further suggests a shared complexity of understanding, a rhetorical "wink" at an audience that is expected to also have mixed feelings about the image, depression, and the lifeworld in which they find themselves. Like the other memes in my sample, this meme is also an example of a meme that uses creativity to "release" suffering through explosive laughter; the punchline seems calculated to provoke laughter at the "crippling depression" in the post (see Figure 5.3).

Figure 5.3

This Post Is Hacked

THIS POST IS
HACKED
ONLY PEOPLE
WITH crippling depression
CANUpvote THIS

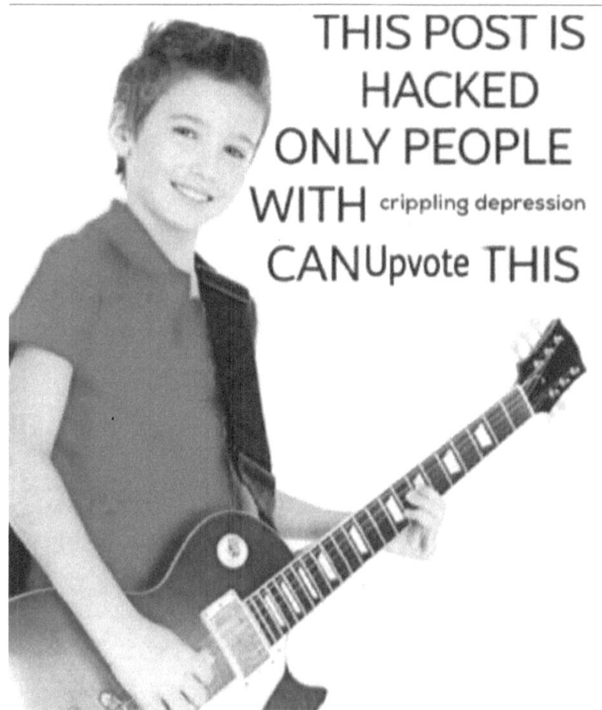

Of course, the irony in the meme in Figure 5.3 is that anyone can upvote it if they choose, furthering the presumption of universal depression. The image itself is slightly "cursed" (i.e., as discussed in Chapter Four), and professes to be "hacked," as the young boy in the picture displays a forced smile. The usage of "crippling" depression underscores a close relationship with suffering, especially given "crippling depression"

and its status as a meme in and of itself. By drawing on the circulatory affective topic of crippling depression, the meme takes a further step by invoking the lifeworld: crippling depression is the understood experience of a daily embodied fight for survival. Upvoting the post marks a tacit recognition of the struggle.

Similarly, Figure 5.4 is an example of the meme trend to meme about depression memes, a kind of meta-joke that often comments on memes' curative powers, which are both "cures" for depression but also ways of avoiding "real" cures and therefore exacerbators of depression through glamorization (as discussed in earlier chapters). Indeed, memes are considered both causes and cures for depression and are discussed as such in the memes themselves (as noted in examples throughout this book and as colloquially discussed both on- and offline). The example in Figure 5.4 utilizes multiple layers of affective and circulatory elements, too numerous to adequately capture. For one, the deer-in-the-headlights look on a *Simpsons* television series character combines reaction images with cultural embeddedness. For another, "I just think they're neat" while holding a noose speaks to multiple complex meme tropes regarding suicide, coping, and graveyard humor online, along with the more obvious connections to pop culture and memes in general.

However, this meme takes the joke a step further, by referring to the online memeworld as a place filled with depression memes, at least according to the punchline. The meme invites the audience into a "club" of depression memes online (while simultaneously self-deprecating their use), then goes one step further by presuming that "everyone" is part of the ambient lifeworld familiar with depression memes. By invoking the (presumably shared) practice of saving a large quantity of depression memes on one's phone, the meme invites the viewer to relate to that same experience of coping (or not coping, as the case may be). Through enthymeme, the meme assumes that the viewer(s) are familiar with the online enclave of depression; by invoking membership in the group, the meme assumes both the existence of the category and the Everyperson's participation in it, culminating in an understanding of the lifeworld as a place to be depressed. By engaging a collective laugh at a human tendency to save non-human reminders of depression, the meme evokes a heightened awareness of humans in collectivity; at the same time, the humans in that collectivity are (apparently) aware of the same types of memes. The ability of the mentioned "friends" to recognize depression memes as a genre further underscores this point, as memes stand in for the ambient "scaffolding" that holds up the world (Rickert, 2013).

Like the material objects discussed previously (such as mugs, t-shirts, and posters), the meme in Figure 5.4 also contains elements of materiality through its various components. The layered noose on top of the screenshot from a television show speaks of a kind of permanence juxtaposed with ephemerality. The human actor/acted-upon that views a meme like this can consider themselves part of a complex web of nooses, tv shows, tv characters, memes, symptoms, and other ambient structural elements, all interacting in a unique moment of blockage at the point where viewer and meme meet. The contrasting verbal and visual elements, too, provide a kind of juxtaposition in mood or flavor, as the mock seriousness of the top part of the meme contrasts with the "lighthearted" bottom section, which nonetheless contains an image of a noose. Instead of merely supposing a "club" (as with the memes in Chapter Four), this meme interacts with the non-material in ways that suggest an ambient relationship with an ambient lifeworld of suffering.

Figure 5.4

1,653 Depression Memes

When your friends ask you why you have 1,653 depression memes saved on your phone
I just think they're neat.

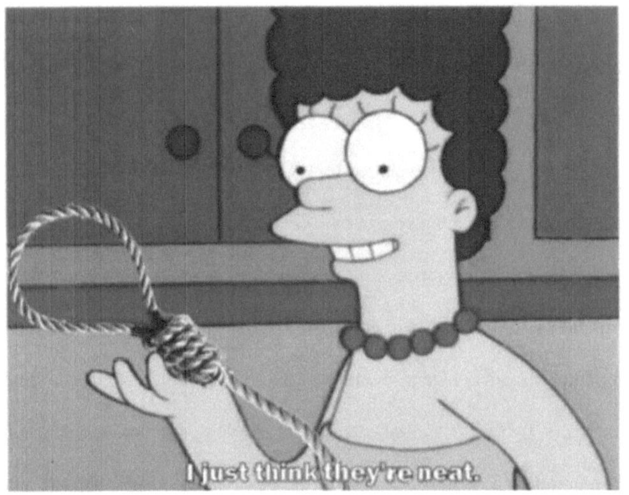

Further, the chaos of the meme/lifeworld is momentarily solidified in the presence of these elements, then released in the laughter of grim humor, another example of blockage and release through humor which points back to Cvetkovich's (2012) claims about the power of art in relieving tensions of depression – which, she says, creates a release of emotional tension through the ritual practice of art. The meme in Figure 5.4 also incorporates other memetic tropes in its layers to participate in the memetic environment of depression. For Rickert (2013), an essential component of ambient rhetoric is "its embodied and embedded or situated character, its dispersal across things that themselves have gradations of agency, and its dynamic emergence within an environment that occasions certain effects," although he clarifies that "to say this is not to deny the existence or importance of intent but rather to insist that within any given rhetorical event, intent cannot suffice for its full accounting as rhetoric" (p. 36).

Other interpretations could be inferred, but more importantly, Figure 5.4 hinges upon a memetic debate about the validity of memes as social markers of depression and the online groups that use them. The punchline hinges on the implied universality of memes as (non)coping mechanisms and suggests a globalized attunement to depression specifically and suffering more generally, especially as diagnosis can only be inferred through context clues. Since "your friends" are asking why "you" have saved the memes, there is a question of diagnosis. Certainly, the meme mentions depression by name, but it also invokes the memetic trope of undiagnosed or undisclosed depression in the caption, coupled with a contradictory assertion about the appropriateness of memes while holding a noose.

In another example, Figure 5.5 invites the viewer to "upvote this [post] to die instantly," a double entendre that "tricks" the viewer into upvoting the meme (giving the poster social clout by making their post more popular) and with the added benefit of a convenient suicide (tongue in cheek). Like the memes in the previous chapters, this meme uses visual/verbal elements to create the joke (it is deliberately minimalist, for one thing), but fails to designate a particular audience. In the spaces between there is an implied "you" unfettered by any human or animal figures. In particular, the meme hinges on the depression meme trope to speak to a general audience; in contrast to the meme above about "only people with crippling depression," this meme makes no qualms about who this meme is "for;" it merely invites participation in anyone who sees it.

Importantly, this meme turns upon an assumption that *everyone* who sees the post wishes to die instantly, and further, will laugh (or not laugh, as the case may be) at the suggestion. Of course, this meme was posted on a sub-Reddit for depression memes, so it is a safe assumption that others on the platform will also experience depression symptoms. This meme, in particular, probably inhabits depression meme pages, rather than the internet more broadly. Further, usage of "upvote" as a term indicates its existence on Reddit, where upvoting is the social currency of the realm. However, this meme is a screencapture – it is not merely a textpost. So, if the original text was posted on Reddit, someone has memed it by reposting it at least once. Still, Poe's Law (Phillips & Milner, 2017) dictates that intents, audiences, and reactions are utterly unpredictable, and the suggestive humor in reaching out to others who might also want to die hints at an attunement toward a widespread empathy with the impulse of death.

Figure 5.5

Upvote This To Die

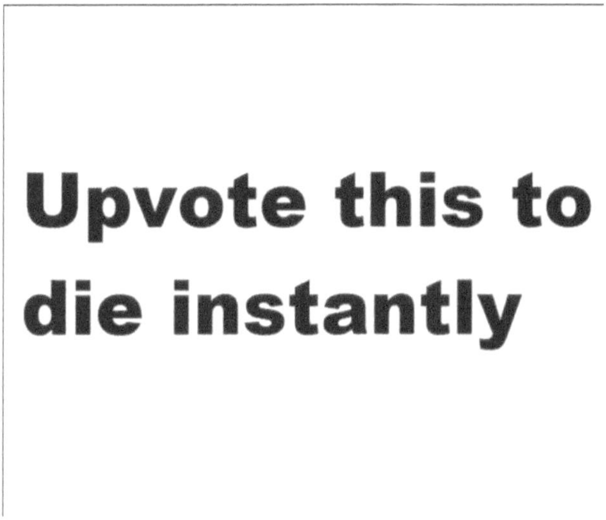

Upvote this to die instantly

Again, this example requires a number of affective and circulatory leaps to "get" the joke. Without context, it makes little sense; the meme presumes intimate familiarity with *topoi* of suicide memes, graveyard humor, depression symptoms, and others. The joke relies on perhaps the greatest presumptive leap out of any of my chosen examples: the presumption that the viewer wishes to die. Moreover, it presumes that the viewer welcomes assistance in dying. Like the examples in the previous chapter, it draws upon circulatory topics of suicide, but from a much more generalized perspective of attunement to suicide.

Similarly, in Figure 5.6, the meme offers advice to the user's social media followers, displaying an attunement to the memetic *topos* of mental health in the holiday season, the small-talk topic of holiday pursuits, and their suitability to one's own mood. The "feeling" of Christmas holds significant sway in many Western cultural contexts and is associated with the innocence of youth and joyful connectivity with family and friends. The grimness of lost innocence permeates a variety of depression memes; this is merely one example of the coming-of-age trope (and several crop up throughout this project). However, Figure 5.5 is illustrative because it speaks to a generalized other that is presumed in need of support during a Christmas season that, to the author, is lacking in something it ought to have: the "happiness" so highly prized in post-modernity (as Ahmed, 2010, might suggest).

For Rickert (2013), "speakers or writers may well understand themselves as working with conscious intent, yet the intention may be causally irrelevant to the effects produced in the audience" (p. 35). That is, regardless of whether a rhetor intends a particular affect or any affect at all, that rhetorical node still joins the rhetorical atmosphere. While Poe's Law (Phillips & Milner, 2017) renders intent problematic, it is also irrelevant: regardless of whether memers "intend" to make particular claims about depression or not, their memes leave traces of rhetoricity not easily detected by the casual observer. The agency working beneath the surface holds as much rhetorical power as any conscious intent to persuade, and in the example of Figure 5.6, the ambivalent affects swirl in a grander sense of a globalized awareness of what it means to "feel like Christmas" (or not to, as the case may be).

Figure 5.6

Doesn't Feel Like Christmas

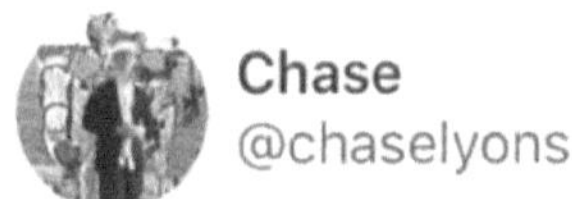

it's not that it "doesn't feel like a Christmas" you just haven't been happy since you were 12

The example in Figure 5.6 draws also heavily on the youth culture trope that pervades many depression memes, as does the example in Figure 5.7, which depicts satisfaction as a reaction to "Depressed teens hearing about WWIII" (see Figure 5.7). The reaction image is that of Kronk, from a popular animated Disney film and often utilized in memes, *The Emperor's New Groove,* underscoring an affective and circulatory dimension of embeddedness in this particular meme. The usage of Kronk as a character highlights a theme tracing all the memes in this chapter; that of ambivalent (un)sympathy with the character.

Memeworlders familiar with the character know that Kronk is an unlikely hero. In the movie, he is portrayed as ignorant, incompetent, and clownish, even while spewing forth painfully obvious logic that even the "smartest" characters in the film fail to grasp.

Kronk's ambivalence as a sympathetic/unsympathetic character is particularly revealing in terms of his "mental deficiencies," which provide punchlines throughout the piece. Though more subtle in some of the other examples in this chapter, Figure 5.7 highlights the delicate question of mental "fitness" playing throughout depression memes, which ambivalently questions the soundness/unsoundness of depression as a perspective of the world.

Further, the trope of "depressed teens" is a common one in memes online, as Gen Zs are purportedly all suicidal memers (at least, according to colloquial accounts found in internet spaces). Again, this meme indicates an awareness of a large body of people ("teens") and their eagerness for global war – not because they wish to participate, but because it is part of a supposed mass suicide plan (the hidden enthymeme in this picture). That is, the meme represents a *Stimmung* of suicide-as-desirable through its juxtaposition of humor and depression. Since the ambient perspective ambience "dissolves the assumed separation between what is (privileged) human doing and what is passively material" (Rickert, 2013, p. 3), depression memes, in particular, provide an example of rhetoric that dissolves material/non-material boundaries, as human and non-human actants participate in a reciprocal creation of memetic tropes.

Figure 5.7

It's All Coming Together

Depressed teens hearing about WWIII :

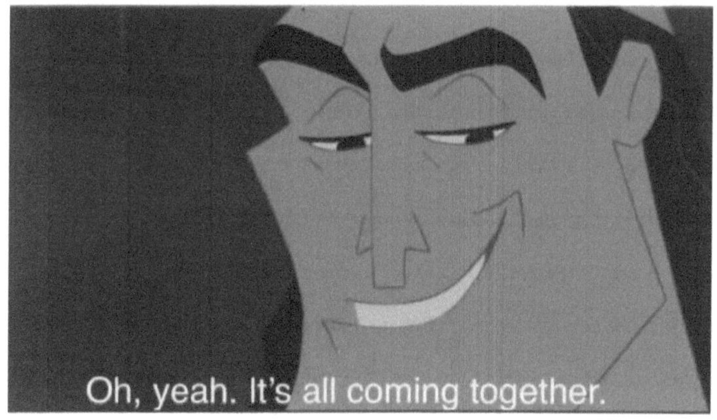

As previously discussed, the process of meme production is primarily through circulation, the element within the larger construct of ambience. By Rickert's (2013) view, rhetoric is an art "buoyed up by" and "delivered over to" ambience. In the case of depression memes, claims made by the memes are buoyed up by and delivered over to the contemporary rhetorical environment. Simultaneously, those memes become part of the contemporary rhetorical environment that then allows and supports more memes. Since "place is not simply an immediate environment; it includes the background by means of which things show up as what they are" (Rickert, 2013, p. 55), memes are exist as part of the scaffolding of a many-layered environment, constantly giving over to new environmental formulations which then produce new memes.

As I argued in Chapter Four, ambivalent affective readings of depression memes provide a picture of the rhetorical universe as one of circulatory affects, or, affects that rely upon circulatory rhetorics of emotion. Depression memes mark one form of rhetorical dwelling that emphasizes both human and non-human interactants while also providing a means to view both meaning and motion. In other words, depression memes are one example of human/nonhuman interaction through these complex systems of bodies, computers, groups, minds, emotions, and other sites of rhetorical environment. The entanglements of environment and self are inextricably linked, and memes are markers of these entanglements. In this way, ambience, as a theory, can illuminate the memeworld as "attunement . . . given in its dynamic unfolding by an originary, worldly rhetoricity, an affectability inherent in how the world comes to be" (Rickert, 2013, p. 8).

In a similar vein, Figure 5.8 capitalizes on that same youth culture by suggesting that "'we're just suicidal kids telling other suicidal kids that suicide isn't the answer.'" The use of "we" here is suggestive, as is the usage of quotation marks, implying that the quote is a significant one and meaningful to a group with some form of solidarity. The origins of the quote are nebulous, as they have been attributed to a secret posted on the Whisper app (a platform designed for anonymous secrets), lyrics sung by a rapper named Royce da 5'9", and poetry posted on Wattpad by username Melancholic_Lotus13, and various other locations online. The origin is of less importance than the sentiment, which has been passed around the internet in dozens of formats since its origin (whatever that origin may be).

Figure 5.8

Just Suicidal Kids

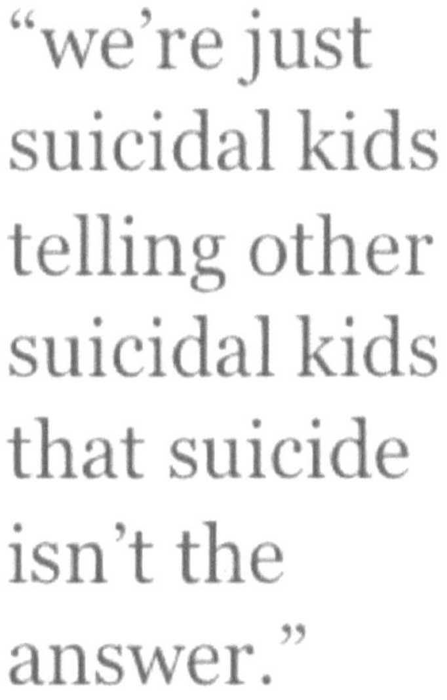

"we're just suicidal kids telling other suicidal kids that suicide isn't the answer."

Like the six-word story about baby shoes I discussed in Chapter Three, the quote in Figure 5.8 has been, by and large, interpreted as sincere (i.e., non-humorously). However, the original author is largely unknown, at least according to my sources (listed above). An original author, in fact, might give the quote less meaning in a discourse that seems to have co-opted the quote as one of solidarity and support. In an ambient environment of suffering, group-ownership of quotes such as this one provides a hazy, yet unified, picture of globalized suicidal tendencies. Indeed, the abundance of suicide references in my sample suggests a certain preoccupation with death, which might be expected as a symptom of depression but feels jarring as a symptom of cultural malaise.

Whether an internet user creates memes or merely views them, engages in sporadic scrolling or habitual, or any other number of permutations, the internet user plays some agential and acted-upon role. As it is not possible to be not in a mood, it is *almost* impossible, these days, to be wholly detached from memes. Regardless of intent, to be an internet user is to be a person connected (however vaguely) with the purview of memes. New media technologies and rhetorics, though seemingly ephemeral, are part of the ambient "carpentry" that reveals and does significant rhetorical work. An example Rickert (2013) uses throughout his seminal text is music, which, as "background noise," actually generates the atmosphere of a rhetorical environment; for Rickert, the new age popularity of ambient music is suggestive, particularly given its name. Technological advances have found increasing ways to play with the environmental capacities of rhetoric, and the advent of ambient music, digital billboards, VR goggles, one-tap payments, driverless cars, QR codes, virtual assistant technologies, and other non-human actors reciprocally influence human interactants.

Humans have always attended to the rhetoricity of environment, even as recent technological advances have made the connection more obvious. In my own experience of sharing, receiving, discussing, and creating memes, my own circulatory spheres are in relationship with me, and I with them, as we all interact in a vast network of affective information. The result is a particular kind of *attunement* toward depression memes—they find me as often as I find them. That attunement is the same sensitivity toward depression that led me to ask: "is everyone depressed?"

Memes, as publicly shared and publicly owned, shingle the rhetorical galaxies of depression. Further, as denizens of the material informational environment, memes are in relationship with the humans they interact with. As actors that take on the invisible subject "you" (as I suggested in Chapter Three), they flip the script on how we can perceive the relationship between rhetoric and rhetor. Then, memes ebb and flow through various positionalities in physical and digital spaces (as I demonstrated in Chapter Four). According to Rickert (2013), "humans and nonhumans—actants of varying agentive weight and value—are threaded through each other and across networks, combining and recombining in flexible assemblages" (p. 24). Online, there are many levels of engagement one can choose from, but all are part of the rhetorical atmosphere.

Throughout this chapter, I have spoken of attunements in the plural. Rickert (2013) concerns himself with attunement generally as his establishment of the concept, but I suggest that ambivalence dictates multiplicities of attunements. As Rickert (2013) outlined, attunement should not be conflated with subjectivity, as "being so entangled, so caught up in the richness of the situation, an attunement is nothing subjective" (Rickert, 2013, p. 9). In other words, "a mood is not something specific that belongs to me first; it is *not* possible *not* to be in a mood" (Ahmed, 2014, p. 14). That is, "mood is not reducible to psychological or conscious cognitive states, to 'interior' phenomena, since it is constitutively entangled within and emerges from the environment in which we are situated and therefore also is a prerequisite for intelligibility as such" (Rickert, 2013, p. 14). Rather, the *Stimmungs* in which we find ourselves are so complex and all-encompassing that we cannot know anything outside of those attunements.

However, Rickert (2013) hastens to clarify that an ambient relationship between humans and non-humans must not "lapse" into "naïve anthropomorphism"; instead, Rickert (2013) invites us to consider Heidegger's fourfold theory of things as a way to understand that "things make claims on us that help constitute not just the various kinds of knowledge we produce but also our very ways of being in the world. Knowledge of the world therefore cannot be partitioned off" (p. 228). Memetic tropes, then, are in partnership with human beings in complex ways.

In other words, we are not merely giving things power: we are acknowledging ourselves as interactants in a world of human and non-human interactants. Indeed, "the word matter refers to issues, relations, import, and knowledge as well [as material objects]" (Rickert, 2013, p. 227), and all must be given due consideration as part of rhetorical atmosphere. Thus, viewing atmosphere as a relationship allows a rendering of individual elements as agential so we can regain agency with the components with which we are in relationship. As these elements blend and merge, separate and conglomerate, we begin to see a picture of depression (literally billions of memetic pictures, actually, scattered throughout an ambient rhetorical atmosphere) that asserts certain ways of knowing and being in the world; these knowings and beings are the "carpentry" within which we can operate (Rickert, 2013).

Our ambient dwelling in suffering is evident in the memes we post; depression has become a public mood in more ways than one. That is, these memes demonstrate an awareness of globalized depression, the assumption that many humans experience depression symptoms, even if the localized self is the one "with" a diagnosis of depression. For instance, another meme suggested that "the human body is 80% water, so we're all just cucumbers with anxiety" (see Appendix C). This meme appeared dutifully with the other memes in my sample, placed among the most popular posts on a sub-Reddit for depression. The inclusion of an anxiety meme on a forum about depression further underscores my point about the permeability of discourses and the generalized suffering found in conversations online. Even on forums that self-profess to be about depression, topical boundaries are loose; conversely, the *topos* of suffering fills and surrounds multiple and varied spaces in the online and offline lifeworld.

Further, the permeability of memes and spaces online and off paints a picture of rhetoric that blurs the boundaries of human and non-human. Memes take on humanness and humans take on memeness as we participate in memes and they participate in us. The lifeworld and the memeworld blend and merge into a conglomerative, ever-shifting *Stimmung* of depression as a post-modern zeitgeist through the ambient worlding of suffering. By suggesting that "we're all just cucumbers with anxiety" (see Appendix C), the meme furthers a global project of inadvertent (almost casual) attunement to suffering; since suffering is trending (through an enthymematic leap), it therefore must be "correct" to suffer with everyone else and to meme about doing so.

The ambivalent, pointed discourses in depression memes interrogate levels of attunement; they seem to ask, "are you aware of my depression?" and, more poignantly, "Are you awake to depression in general?" Many of the memes in the sample seem to suggest a necessity of being "woke" to the vicissitudes of mental health in the digital era. Although awareness is considered an integral part of activism, I caution that a more mindful usage of awareness might be more meaningful, at least in online spaces. Depression memes, it seems, can provide powerful releases of tensioned symptoms, but can also serve as pulpits for depression symptoms hidden as debonair revelations of universal suffering. The countless homages to depression on t-shirts, mugs, memes, and other material and non-material rhetorics suggest an eager acceptance of depressive tropes. Although perhaps a meaningful release for individual sufferers, the collective #mood is perhaps one to re-consider.

As another way to describe how ambience functions, Rickert (2013) likened it to Plato's *chōra,* "an ancient attempt to think the relation between matter and activity, work and space, background and meaning, and thus it already starts to broach issues concerning relations among bodies, minds, and world" (p. 42). The *chōra,* as in the theatrical chorus that provided background narration in ancient dramatic performances, "is crucial for bringing life to otherwise static and overly bound conceptions of world and activity" (Rickert, 2013, p. 42). Memes, in this case, provide a background chorus of angst, a #mood that is set by the blended voices setting the global post-modern scene.

If the *chōra* represented ambience in ancient times, technological advances have facilitated an ever-increasing ability to interact with non-human entities in increasingly meaningful ways. Now, suggests Rickert (2013), "we are entering an age of ambience, one in which boundaries between subject and object, human and nonhuman, and information and matter dissolve" (p. 1). Like the background narration of the Greek chorus, memes provide an unbound commentary on bound "conceptions of world" (Rickert, 2013, p. 32). Indeed, "technologies of all kinds, media related and otherwise, are themselves becoming ambient, not only as scaffolding for our everyday activities, but as material actants affecting us through behind-the-scenes programming, including decisioning algorithms" (Rickert, 2013, p. 44). Memes, I suggest, are useful examples of a technology that provides a *chōra* of suffering via circulatory globules of affect online.

As affect studies critiques the necessity of Cartesian dualism, so does an ambient perspective, because it suggests that human attunements cannot be canted or corked; depression is not a definable experience and rhetorical attunements cannot be measured via empirical means. The ineffability of human experience as circulated online superimposes our dwelling-place(s), which merge and separate in meeting-places of release and blockage. Our "way of being there with one another," by design, revels in vagaries and imprecisions that allow authentic, rather than accurate, depictions of *Stimmung,* a rhetorical project that can be undertaken at the individual and global level. Memes are one way that an individual can participate in this endeavor, should they so choose. The ambient particles of the rhetorical atmosphere (in memes and otherwise) paper the walls of our dwelling places; it is up to us to notice.

Conclusion

Western empiricism would suggest that to escape the influence of worldview in favor of accurate portrayals of experience is not only necessary, but also desirable; ambience would suggest that it is neither possible nor worthwhile. For Rickert (2013), "mood/attunement is not 'inside' us, although neither is it simply exterior; rather, it is 'the way of our being there with one another'" (p. 146). The notion of "interior" dispositions, so entangled with external temperaments, is especially crucial in a topic like depression; although depression memes ostensibly describe the "inner" mental and emotional states of human subjects, those inner states of being are so embroiled in outer states of being that it is virtually impossible to separate them.

My own attunements (as opposed to subjectivities) throughout my exploration of ambient rhetoric has taken place as part of grander "moods" of depression, memes, rhetoric, academic writing, and other ambient structures; my subjectivity, rather than merely influencing my project, has been a by-product of larger attunements in the lifeworld. Although I have owned my attunements (described clumsily in terms of subjectivities) throughout, my own attunements can never fully be set forth in writing in any satisfactory way. Likewise, my readership is already subject to attunements that have colored individual readings of this project. A fully authentic chronical of attunement would incorporate affective, historical, mental, relational, and other ambivalent dimensions of experience; attunement is simply too vast to "pin down" to any self-imposed quest for so-called "accuracy." Like the ineffable experience of suffering, attunement is inexpressible; and yet, both can be explored through attending to the molecules of rhetorical atmosphere(s).

Chapter 6: Conclusion

On internet spaces, social media users participate in "signal boosts" to support popular causes (Signal-boost, 2020). A signal boost is a concerted effort to post, upvote, like, and share information about social movements, awareness campaigns, or even re-framings of salient, widespread cultural beliefs. A signal boost, then, is a deliberate attunement to particular ideas by drawing attention to them in online spaces through circulation. Although signal boosts are deliberate attempts to promote a topic using the same principles outlined here, perhaps a similar process occurs through inadvertent signal boosting of depression memes online. Throughout this book, I have attuned the reader to the subtle, affective, enthymematic *topos* of depression that permeates our social world, particularly online but also in material-world spaces. Memes have been my subject matter, although a variety of rhetorical texts would have sufficed; and yet, memes provided an efficient and impactful example that are highly self-aware of the discourses they portray.

As cited early in the first chapter of this book, Czyzewski (2001) noted an interesting paradox; although post-modernity supposedly freed us from a variety of pre-modern cultural evils, post-modern citizens perceive these same evils as increasing at an alarming rate, despite post-modernity's promise of freedom from them. How, then, are we to understand the difficulties we now face, since post-modernity has "saved" us from pre-modern suffering? In a treatise on positivity in post-modernity, Ahmed (2010) writes about the association between happiness and appropriateness: "If we are happy, then we are well; or we have done well … The association between wellness and feeling can be powerful" (p. 199). That is, in post-modern times, to be happy is to be acceptable; to be unhappy is inappropriate (Ahmed, 2010). However, as I have demonstrated throughout, ambivalence provides a more authentic portrayal of the experience of depression, which Ahmed (2010) affirms in her exploration of the false "promise" of happiness in post-modernity. For Ahmed, happiness is an impossible injunction that post-modern citizens ultimately fail to achieve, due to the false hope of perfect happiness all the time.

In this conclusion, I outline the tensions extant in the global scaffolding of depression memes as proposed throughout and relate them to the broader usage of attunement as theory and praxis. In a time of global reporting on widespread trouble and strife, rhetorics of suffering color the rhetorical landscape filled with ever-present and immediate discourses of suffering. Throughout this book, I have sought to contextualize depression memes as ambient building blocks in the rhetorical background of post-modernity. In Chapter Three, I explored the intricacies of individualized diagnosis as contrasted with generalized suffering, displayed through affective enthymemes that made the ineffable, effable. In Chapter Four, I built upon solitary memes as parts of grander circulatory cultures, noting their ability to release "blockages" through the outlet of humor. Then, I explored the global attunement to the universal suffering of the human condition, as evidenced by the attunement to suffering found in the memes in my sample (Chapter Five). Overall, I have used my own attunement to depression memes as a lens through which to propose a particular orientation toward depression that permeates the post-modern culturescape. As the "big sad" or "big mood" online, depression is woven through the cultural tapestry of post-modern life in several tensioned ways.

First, an ambivalent reading of depression memes as attunement acknowledges their problematic ability to "signal boost" suffering, which, conversely, also provide salutary avenues for re-framing, release of emotional blockage, and opened dialogues surrounding how we might understand and ameliorate mental illness, both online and off. Specifically, Cvetkovich (2012) argues for a cultural view of depression as an alternative to contemporary discourses on depression, which, she suggests, foreground medical explanations and treatments to the detriment of significant social factors and fail to fully assist those in need of help. As post-modern tidbits of activism, depression memes similarly place the impetus for depression "in life," or in "the big sad," rather than in the depressed individual. For Cvetkovich, this is a freeing realization; it removes the "fault" of mental illness from the internal and moves it to the external, at least in part. By viewing depression as a public feeling, Cvetkovich's perspective allows individual ownership over the social injustices human beings face every day through expression, which she views as a "spiritual" practice of connection-seeking and activism for underprivileged populations.

Sexism, racism, classism, and other political disempowerments bind and oppress individuals in real and meaningful ways largely ignored by the preferred psychological explanation favored by capitalistic pharmaceutical monoliths. Social factors, Cvetkovich (2012) argues, have been undervalued by medical interpretations of depression, whose "social construction of depression is a theoretical premise that is only the beginning of a complex story" (p. 100). Women, people of color, and LGBTQA folks, in particular, are often told their depression is not real, while privileged individuals can rely exclusively on their symptoms as evidence for receiving assistance. McRobbie (2009), in her chapter on post-feminist disorders, drew on the works of Judith Butler and Michel Foucault to demonstrate the "normative pathology" surrounding disordered eating, mood disorders, self-harm, and other mental health concerns. For underserved people, to be ill is "normal," and assistance suffers accordingly (McRobbie, 2009). When memes critique these powerful discourses, they create both a disruption of harmful discourses even while "boosting" the existence of these harmful discourses through affective expression.

Secondly, depression memes provide social support and healing through connection by inviting users into an online "club" of depression. On the other hand, this "club" has a tendency to normalize illness "behaviors" (whether or not they are genuine markers of illness) by inviting others to participate in memetic tropes—such as saying "mood" when faced with struggles, both large and small. By connecting with someone beyond the self, memes provide a bursting of pent-up affects that circulate and congregate and clog up the doorways of the lifeworld; through infinitesimal releases of emotion via laughter, memes serve as micro-clearings of the blockages found in the daily workings of cultural malaise. And yet, this same circulation has a tendency to "move" pieces of depression through social groups, encouraging permeability. According to Brennan's (2004) depiction of the affective permeability between human beings (and, Rickert would add, non-human beings), moving affects through social groups have consequences, as these circulations encourage the positive and negative normalization of mental illness "behaviors" (genuine or otherwise).

As a partial (albeit limited) solution, Cvetkovich's (2012) suggestion to view depression as a "public feeling" invites us to consider the sociocultural aspects of depression and critique our own privileges regarding them. Similarly, depression memes, in a self-aware manner, refer to the "big sad" and openly deplore the normalization of depression (and other mental illnesses) online. Research and online discussion on eating disorder blogs echoes this charge by considering the tensioned powers of social support in these spaces (Brotsky & Giles, 2007; Burke, 2012; Curry & Ray, 2010; Custers & Van den Bulck, 2009; Haas, Irr, Jennings & Wagner, 2010; Knapton, 2013; Lipczynska, 2007; Riley, Rodham, & Gavin, 2009). Perhaps these discourses (along with depression memes) are also normalizing *suffering,* which has significant rhetorical consequences. Thus, hyper-medicalized discourses allow the normalization of psychological disorders by failing to acknowledge the significant cultural, social, and discursive factors involved, but opening discussion about the complex nature of what it means to be a human in post-modernity.

Thirdly, memes are viral discursive markers of contemporary attunements to depression, symptoms, and suffering, which creates a tension between de-escalating stigma and escalating glamorization. By attuning viewers to particular lifeworlds, they invite us into new understandings of those lifeworlds, which may or may not be beneficial to the viewers own mental health. While they use symptoms imprecisely, memes favor Cvetkovich's (2012) description of depression, which she calls "daily lives that are pervaded by a combination of anxiety and numbness" (p. 1). Cvetkovich's depiction of depression as a globalized, politicized, and collective experience serves as a counterpoint to the stigmatized, hyper-medicalized viewpoint of mental illness, which tends to blame the individual for their mental illness while simultaneously questioning its existence (as is critiqued in meme examples throughout).

At the same time, memes provide relief from suffering through creative expression, which Cvetkovich (2012) calls a "form of spiritual experience" that connects the individual to something beyond the self, a globalized awareness of connectivity (p. 192). Although she explores several forms of creative expression in her work, she emphasizes writing as a meaningful practice to alleviate some of the cultural "dis-ease" that is depression. As a spiritual practice, she suggests, writing:

> ties to the ordinary and the repetitive and its fragile and ephemeral presence in places where feelings of despair and hopelessness are also powerfully present suggest that it is not necessarily a form of transcendence or escape from the messy realities of the here and now. (p. 197)

By Cvetkovich's estimation, creative expression alleviates depression because it is a release from when affects become "too much," a suggestion that, I suggest, parallels Edwards' (2011) reference to *hisa* (chaos) and *zhama* (blockage): when the chaos threatens to overwhelm, creative release allows the excess to dissipate into the rhetorical atmosphere. Just as the colloquial definitions of memes as a "cure" for depression suggest, memetic expression can provide a similar release of blockages online (albeit an ambivalent one). By questioning the discourses surrounding life, death, therapy, treatment, illness, and wellness, depression memes criticize the mainstream, pharmaceutical viewpoint of depression, partly through humorous one-upmanship (or down, as the case may be) and partly through turning prominent discourses upside down.

Perhaps, then, memes serve as pockets of creative expression that provide a release of blockage while simultaneously re-assembling the same scattered pieces of depression permeating the discourse. Examples throughout the internet aver that memes are "cures" for depression, even while those same discourses express concern at the glamorizing power of those same memes. Taken singly, they represent particles in a grand interplay of tension and release; taken together, they provide a picture of current beliefs around what it means to be a depressed person and what it means to be a human being in post-modernity. In so doing, however, depression memes can conflate these two concepts, suggesting that clinical depression is overblown because we're all suffering in post-modernity. Thus, even though I find value in depression memes' use of humor to point to social contributions to suffering, I do so with ambivalence because (1) individuals do suffer from clinical depression and (2) depression memes can belittle this experience with their humor.

Memes, somehow, are at the center; they are daily-use rhetorical expressions that partly relieve, partly re-affirm, the vague, low-level throb of unease that underpins post-modernity. The experience of depression is often rendered ineffable by the clinical nature of diagnosed symptoms, which are, in turn, rendered effable by memes, which then re-enter the public discourse of depression and further normalize the experience (and the process repeats). By insisting upon ubiquitous depression, memes both de-stigmatize and re-stigmatize salient issues at the heart of mental health discourses today by attuning their viewers to particular ambient lifeworlds. As such, the internet collective seems hyper-aware of the effects of the trendiness of depression, and yet seems in no hurry to change; in a complex tension of memes, their messages, and their movements, "Everyone" seems aware, but no one seems to know what to make of it. In other words, the "deep" rhetoric of suffering saturates the "molecules" of rhetorical atmospheres, which play an "active role . . . in human development, dwelling, and culture" (Rickert, 2013, p. 3).

This deep rhetoric, or attunement, it seems, is deeply entrenched; indeed, "we cannot simply and directly choose to dwell otherwise" (Rickert, 2013, p. 239). Should we wish to adjust the sails of our attunement, Rickert (2013) suggests, "a new attunement is necessary, one that will spring from preparatory work across the full range of human dwelling, and this attunement must ring the fourfold if it is to grip us sufficiently to awaken us" (p. 239). That is, "there can be no simple revaluing without deeper transformations in our lived relations to the world in ways that in turn attune us differently to world, that is, that bring the world as world to us otherwise than it now is for us" (Rickert, 2013, p. 239). However, must we always assume that new attunement is necessary? The complex debate about depression, memes, normalization, and medicalization suggests a variety of ambivalent affects associated with joking about suffering online, many of which could bring about reduced stigma, relief of symptoms (through rhetorical expression), or even new dialogues for social improvements regarding mental illness. While depression memes perhaps normalize mental illness, they also critique social discourses of depression and might minimize the daily lived individual experience of clinical depression. Perhaps humans have always joked about depression; maybe depression memes are unique only by their permanence in online spaces. However, the durability of the internet allows for a certain complexity not available to other formats, meaning that humanity is learning to joke about depression in increasingly intricate ways.

When I discuss my research with undergraduates, they invariably know exactly what I am talking about and begin discussing their own examples from a variety of platforms, enthusiastically cataloguing the relatability of internet memes and depression, as well as deploring the glamor of depression online. Some have told me that their therapists have begun using memes (as in the examples in Chapter One) as talking points to help open up difficult topics. The generational, cultural, political, and other socio-cultural gaps extant in contemporary Western culture must be more carefully explored if humanity seeks a more compassionate viewpoint for mental health. Instead of viewing suffering as an internal, individualized weakness, individuals, scholars, and collectives must begin to re-frame discourses of suffering to open new channels of discussion surrounding post-modern suffering and its consequences—memes are an excellent place to start.

Since rhetoric acclimates us to particular attunements, we can interrogate our cultural attunements toward depression and other integral human conditions. By examining our own attunements toward race, class, education, government, ethics, the environment, and other material realities, we can perhaps shift our mechanisms of alignment for the betterment of these material realities. Understanding post-modernity's undercurrent of suffering as depicted through internet memes provides a window into a broader cultural malaise and has relevance to discourses of personhood (and non-personhood). We must interrogate these discourses if humanity seeks a more equitable social paradigm in coming days, as cultural “dis-ease” does not affect everyone equally. Individual choice must step in as the mechanism through which we navigate attunements as the carpentry of our daily life; fine-tuning our own attunements and their signal-boosting capacities might be the first step.

References

Ahmed, S. (2004a). Affective economies. *Social Text, 22*(2), 117–139. 10.1215/01642472-22-2_79-117

Ahmed, S. (2004b). *The cultural politics of emotion*. Edinburgh University Press.

Ahmed, S. (2010). *The promise of happiness*. Duke University Press.

Ahmed, S. (2014). Not in the mood. *New Formations,* 84, 13-22. 0.3898/NeWF.82.01.2014

Akram, U., Drabble, J., Cau, G., Hershaw, F., Rajenthran, A., Lowe, M., Trommelen, C., & Ellis, J. G. (2020). Exploratory study on the role of emotion regulation in perceived valence, humour, and beneficial use of depressive internet memes in depression. *Scientific Reports*, *10*(1). 10.1038/s41598-020-57953-4

Alston, J.P. & Platt, L.A. (1969). Religious humor: A longitudinal content analysis of cartoons. *Sociological Analysis*, *30*(4), 217. 10.2307/3710511

American Psychiatric Association. (2013). *Diagnostic and statistical manual of mental disorders* (5th ed.). Washington, DC.

Andalibi, N., Ozturk, P., & Forte, A. (2017). Sensitive self-disclosures, responses, and social support on Instagram: The case of #depression. *Proceedings of the 2017 ACM Conference on Computer Supported Cooperative Work and Social Computing*, 1485–1500. https://doi.org/10.1145/2998181.2998243

Ask, K., & Abidin, C. (2018). My life is a mess: Self-deprecating relatability and collective identities in the memification of student issues. *Information, Communication & Society*, *21*(6), 834–850. 10.1080/1369118X.2018.1437204

Aune, D. E. (2003). The use and abuse of the enthymeme in New Testament scholarship. *New Testament Studies*, *49*(3), 299–320. 10.1017/S0028688503000146

Bacon, J. (2007). ''Acting as freemen'': Rhetoric, race, and reform in the debate over colonization in *Freedom's Journal*, 1827–1828. *Quarterly Journal of Speech*, *93*(1), 58-83. 10.1080/00335630701326860

Berrios, G. E., & Marková, I. S. (2017). The cultural history of depression. In C. Foster & J. Herring (Eds.), *Depression: Law and ethics.* (pp. 45–57). Oxford University Press.

Bitzer, L. (1968). The rhetorical situation. *Philosophy & Rhetoric, 1*(1), 1-14.

Blackmore, S. J. (1999). *The meme machine*. Oxford University Press.

Boepple, L., Ata, R. N., Rum, R., & Thompson, J. K. (2016). Strong is the new skinny: A content analysis of fitspiration websites. *Body Image*, *17*(2), 132–135. 10.1016/j.bodyim.2016.03.001

Brennan, T. (2004). *The transmission of affect.* Cornell University Press.

Brotsky, S. R., & Giles, D. (2007). Inside the "Pro-ana" community: A covert online participant observation. *Eating Disorders*, *15*(2), 93-109. 10.1080/10640260701190600

Brown, C. & Jasper, K. (1993). *Consuming passions: Feminist approaches to weight preoccupation and eating disorders.* Second Story Press.

Budanovic, N. (2017, October 25). "For sale, baby shoes, never worn": Tracing the history of the shortest story ever told. Retrieved September 30, 2020, from https://www.thevintagenews.com/2017/09/24/for-sale-baby-shoes-never-worn-tracing-the-history-of-the-shortest-story-ever-told/

Burke, E. (2012). Reflections on the waif. *Australian Feminist Studies*, *27*(71), 37-54. 10.1080/08164649.2012.648258

BuzzfeedVideo. (2020). *I accidentally became a meme: Overly attached girlfriend.* YouTube. Retrieved from https://www.youtube.com/watch?v=Elhoa_MIyhw

Carey, J. W. (2009). A cultural approach to communication. In J. W. Carey (Ed.), *Communication as culture: Essays on media and society* (pp. 36-45). New York: Routledge.

Cannizzaro, S. (2016). Internet memes as internet signs: A semiotic view of digital culture. *Sign Systems Studies, 44*(4), 562-586. 10.12697/SSS.2016.44.4.05

Chandler, C. (2015). Memes, enthymemes, and the reproduction of ideology. *Medium.* Retrieved February 12, 2020, from http://currychandler.com/cool-medium/2015/9/14/memes-enthymemes-and-the-reproduction-of-ideology

Chen, K. W. (2018). The internet political meme as remediation of the political cartoon. In A. Sover (Ed.) *The languages of humor: Verbal, visual, and physical humor* (pp. 202-224). London: Bloomsbury.

Chen, W. (2019). A study on the network catchphrases from the perspective of memetics. *Journal of Language Teaching & Research, 10*(1), 190. 10.17507/jltr.1001.21

Collins, M. (2015). The enthymeme: An analysis of sexist advice animals. *Young Scholars in Writing, 12*, 94-103. Retrieved from youngscholarsinwriting.org

Coker, C. (2008). War, memes and memeplexes. *International Affairs*, *84*(5), 903–914. 10.1111/j.1468-2346.2008.00745.x

Corbitt-Hall, D. J., Gauthier, J. M., & Troop-Gordon, W. (2019). Suicidality disclosed online: Using a simulated Facebook task to identify predictors of support giving to friends at risk of self-harm. *Suicide & Life-Threatening Behavior*, *49*(2), 598–613. 10.1111/sltb.12461

Cos, G., & Martin, K. N. (2013). The rhetoric of the hanging chair: Presence, absence, and visual argument in the 2012 presidential campaign. *American Behavioral Scientist*, *57*(12), 1688–1703. 10.1177/0002764213490694

Cronkhite, G. L. (1966). The Enthymeme as Deductive Rhetorical Argument. *Western Speech*, *30*(2), 129–134.

Curry, J., & Ray, S. (2010). Starving for support: How women with anorexia receive 'thinspiration' on the internet. *Journal Of Creativity In Mental Health*, *5*(4), 358-373. 10.1080/15401383.2010.527788

Cursed Image. (2020, September 25). Know Your Meme. Retrieved September 28, 2020, from https://knowyourmeme.com/memes/cursed-image

Curtin, S. C. & Heron, M. (2019). Death rates due to suicide and homicide among persons aged 10–24: United States, 2000–2017. *NCHS Data Report, 352*, 8.

Custers, K., & Van den Bulck, J. (2009). Viewership of pro-anorexia websites in seventh, ninth and eleventh graders. *European Eating Disorders Review*, *17*(3), 214-219. 10.1002/erv.910

Cvetkovich, A. (2012). *Depression: A public feeling.* Durham: Duke University Press.

Czyzewski, M. (2001). "The anxieties of our times" as a *topos* in public discourse. *Polish Sociological Review, 135*(3), 261–280. Retrieved from https://www.jstor.org/stable/i40057482

Deighton-Smith, N., & Bell, B. T. (20170511). Objectifying fitness: A content and thematic analysis of #fitspiration images on social media. *Psychology of Popular Media Culture*, *7*(4), 467-483. 10.1037/ppm0000143

Depression Humor. (2020). LookHuman. *My life is a Cat-astrophe T-Shirts.* Retrieved from https://www.lookhuman.com/design/377686-my-life-is-a-cat-astrophe/3600-black-lg.

Depression Meme. (2020). RedBubble. Retrieved from https://www.redbubble.com/shop/?query=depression+meme.

Depression Mugs. (2020). TeePublic. Retrieved from https://www.teepublic.com/mug?query=depression.

Dyck, E. (2002). Topos and enthymeme. *Rhetorica: A Journal of the History of Rhetoric, 20*(2), 105–117. 10.1525/rh.2002.20.2.105

Dynel, M. (2016). "I has seen image macros!" Advice animal memes as visual-verbal jokes. *International Journal of Communication*, *10*(1), 660–668. Retrieved from ijoc.org/index.php/ijoc/article/view/4101

Edbauer, J. (2005). Unframing models of public distribution: From rhetorical situation to rhetorical ecologies. *Rhetoric Society Quarterly, 35*(4), 5–24. 10.1080/02773940509391320

Edwards, B. T. (2011). Tahrir: Ends of circulation. *Public Culture, 23*(3), 493–504. 10.1215/08992363-1336372.

Edwards, D. W. (2016). *Writing in the flow: Assembling tactical rhetorics in an age of viral circulation.* [Doctoral book, Miami University].

Finnegan, C. A., & Kang, J. (2004). "Sighting" the public: Iconoclasm and public sphere theory. *Quarterly Journal of Speech, 90*(4), 377–402. 10.1080/0033563042000302153

Flick, C. (2016). Informed consent and the Facebook emotional manipulation study. *Research Ethics, 12*(1), 14–28. https://doi.org/10.1177/1747016115599568

Flowers, A. A., & Young, C. L. (2010). Parodying Palin: How Tina Fey's visual and verbal impersonations revived a comedy show and impacted the 2008 election. *Journal of Visual Literacy, 29*(1), 47–67. 10.1080/23796529.2010.11674673

Fredal, J. (2018). Is the enthymeme a syllogism? *Philosophy & Rhetoric, 51*(1), 24. 10.5325/philrhet.51.1.0024

Fowler, J. H., & Christakis, N. A. (2008). Dynamic spread of happiness in a large social network: Longitudinal analysis over 20 years in the Framingham Heart Study. *BMJ, 337*(dec04 2), a2338–a2338. https://doi.org/10.1136/bmj.a2338

Friedan, B. (1963). *The feminine mystique.* W. W. Norton & Company.

Gallagher, V. J., & Zagacki, K. S. (2007). Visibility and rhetoric: Epiphanies and transformations in the *Life* photographs of the Selma marches of 1965. *Rhetoric Society Quarterly, 37*(2), 113–135. 10.1080/02773940601016056

Gaonkar, D. P., & Povinelli, E. A. (2003). Technologies of public forms: Circulation, transfiguration, recognition. *Public Culture, 15*(3), 385–398. 10.1215/08992363-15-3-385.

Gries, L. E. (2013). Iconographic tracking: A digital research method for visual rhetoric and circulation studies. *Computers and Composition, 30*(4), 332–348. 10.1016/j.compcom.2013.10.006

Gries, L. E., & Brooke, C.G. (Eds.) (2018). *Circulation, writing, and rhetoric*. Logan: Utah State University Press. 10.2307/j.ctt21668mb.

Grundlingh, L. (2018). Memes as speech acts. *Social Semiotics*, *28*(2), 147–168. 10.1080/10350330.2017.1303020

Haas, S. M, Irr, M. E., Jennings, M. A & Wagner, L. M. (2010). Communicating thin: A grounded model of online negative enabling support groups in the pro-anorexia movement. *New Media and Society, 13*(1) 40–57 10.1177/1461444810363910

Hahner, L. A. (2013). The riot kiss: Framing memes as visual argument. *Argumentation and Advocacy*, *49*(3), 151–166. 10.1080/00028533.2013.11821790

Hale, B. J. (2019). Responding to depression-related Imgur posts: A content analysis of social support and non-bona fide features in user-generated comments. *Digital Health, 5*(1), 1-12. 10.1177/2055207619890476

Hancock, J. T., Gee, K., Ciaccio, K., & Lin, J. M.-H. (2008). I'm sad you're sad: Emotional contagion in CMC. *Proceedings of the ACM 2008 Conference on Computer Supported Cooperative Work - CSCW '08*, 295-298. https://doi.org/10.1145/1460563.1460611

Harold, C. (2004). Pranking rhetoric: 'Culture jamming' as media activism. *Critical Studies in Media Communication, 21*(3): 189–211. doi:10.1080/0739318042000212693

Harvey, A. M., Thompson, S., Lac, A., & Coolidge, F. L. (2019). Fear and derision: A quantitative content analysis of provaccine and antivaccine internet memes. *Health Education & Behavior*, *46*(6), 1012–1023. 10.1177/1090198119866886

Hedegaard, H., Curtin, S. C., & Warner, M. (2020). Increase in suicide mortality in the United States, 1999–2018. *NCHS Data Brief, 362*, 1-8.

Hegde, R. (2010). Eyeing new publics: Veiling and the performance of civic visibility. In D. C. Brouwer & R. Asen (Eds.), *Public modalities: Rhetoric, culture, media, and the shape of public life* (pp. 154-172). Tuscaloosa: University of Alabama Press.

Hill, K. (2014, September 3). Forbes. *Facebook manipulated 689,003 users' emotions for science*. https://www.forbes.com/sites/kashmirhill/2014/06/28/facebook-manipulated-689003-users-emotions-for-science/.

Horowitz, J.M., & Graf, N. (2019). Most U.S. teens see anxiety, depression as major problems. *Pew Research Center's Social & Demographic Trends Project.* Retrieved from https://www.pewsocialtrends.org/2019/02/20/most-u-s-teens-see-anxiety-and-depression-as-a-major-problem-among-their-peers/

Huntington, H. E. (2016). Pepper spray cop and the American dream: Using synecdoche and metaphor to unlock internet memes' visual political rhetoric. *Communication Studies*, *67*(1), 77–93. 10.1080/10510974.2015.1087414

Huntington, H. E. (2017). The affect and effect of internet memes: Assessing perceptions and influence of online user-generated political discourse as media. [Doctoral book, Colorado State University].

Jackson, S. W. (2008). A history of melancholia and depression. In E. R. Wallace IV & J. Gach (Eds.), *History of psychiatry and medical psychology: With an epilogue on psychiatry and the mind-body relation.* (pp. 443–460). Springer.

Jansen, L. (2007). Aristotle's *categories*. *Topoi 26*(1), 153–158. 10.1007/s11245-006-9009-1

Jadayel, R., Medlej, K., & Jadayel, J. J. (2017). Mental disorders: A glamorous attraction on social media? *Journal of Teaching and Education, 7*(1). 465–475. Retrieved from www.universitypublications.net/jte/0701/pdf/V7NA374.pdf

Jenkins, E. S. (2014). The modes of visual rhetoric: Circulating memes as expressions. *Quarterly Journal of Speech, 100*(4), 442–466. 10.1080/00335630.2014.989258

Jennings, K. (2018). *Planet funny: How comedy took over our culture*. Scribner.

Knapton, O. (2013). Pro-anorexia: Extensions of ingrained concepts. *Discourse & Society, 24*(4), 461-477. 10.1177/0957926513482067

Karp, D. A. (1994). Living with depression: Illness and identity turning points. *Qualitative Health Research, 4*(1), 6–30.

Karp, D. A. (2017). *Speaking of sadness: Depression, disconnection, and the meanings of illness*. Oxford University Press.

Katz, Y., & Shifman, L. (2017). Making sense? The structure and meanings of digital memetic nonsense. *Information, Communication & Society, 20*(6), 825–842. 10.1080/1369118X.2017.1291702

Kennerly, M. J., & Pfister, D. S. (2018). Poiēsis, genesis, mimēsis: Toward a less selfish genealogy of memes. In M. J. Kennerly & D. S. Pfister (Eds.) *Ancient rhetorics and digital networks* (pp. 205-228). University of Alabama Press.

Kramer, P. D. (2006). *Against depression.* Penguin Books.

Kochin, M. (2009). From argument to assertion. *Argumentation, 23*(3), 387–396.

Lawlor, C. (2012). *From melancholia to prozac: A history of depression.* Oxford University Press.

Lee, B., & LiPuma, E. (2002). Cultures of circulation: The imaginations of modernity. *Public Culture, 14*(1), 191–213. Retrieved from http://www.wcas.northwestern.edu/projects/globalization/secure/articles/14.1lee.pdf

Leissner, O. (1998). The problem that has no name. *Cardozo Women's Law Journal, 4*(2), 321-408.

Lipczynska, S. (2007). Discovering the cult of Ana and Mia: A review of pro-anorexia websites. *Journal of Mental Health, 16*(4), 545-548. 10.1080/09638230701482402

Lloyd, K. (2013). Reinterpreting enthymemes to include the nonverbal, *JAC, 33*(3), 732-749. Retrieved from https://www.jstor.org/stable/43854576

Lydecker, J. A., Cotter, E. W., Palmberg, A. A., Simpson, C., Kwitowski, M., White, K., & Mazzeo, S. E. (2016). Does this Tweet make me look fat? A content analysis of weight stigma on Twitter. *Eating and weight disorders - studies on anorexia, bulimia and obesity*, *21*(2), 229–235. 10.1007/s40519-016-0272-x

Macagno, F., & Damele, G. (2013). The dialogical force of implicit premises. Presumptions in enthymemes. *Informal Logic*, *33*(3), 41-53. 10.22329/il.v33i3.3679

Machin, D., & Mayr, A. (2012). *How to do critical discourse analysis: A multimodal introduction.* SAGE Publications.

Marshall, J. (2001). Cyber-space, or cyber-topos: The creation of online space. *Social Analysis: The International Journal of Anthropology*, *45*(1), 81–102. Retrieved from https://www.jstor.org/stable/23169992

McCulloch, A. M. (2006). Depression and its expression: Art as problem solver. *International Journal of the Humanities*, *3*(7), 155–162

McLuhan, M. (1968). *War and peace in the global village: An inventory of some of the current spastic situations that could be eliminated by more feedforward*. Bantam Books.

McRobbie, A. (2009). *The aftermath of feminism: Gender, culture and social change*. Sage.

Meyer, W. J., Morrison, P., Lombardero, A., Swingle, K., & Campbell, D. G. (2016). College students' reasons for depression nondisclosure in primary care. *Journal of College Student Psychotherapy*, *30*(3), 197–205.

Michikyan, M. (2020) Depression symptoms and negative online disclosure among young adults in college: A mixed-methods approach. *Journal of Mental Health, 29*(4), 92-400. 10.1080/09638237.2019.1581357

Miguel, E. M., Chou, T., Golik, A., Cornacchio, D., Sanchez, A. L., DeSerisy, M., & Comer, J. S. (2017). Examining the scope and patterns of deliberate self-injurious cutting content in popular social media. *Depression & Anxiety*, *34*(9), 786–793. 10.1002/da.22668

Miller, A. B., & Bee, J. D. (1972). Enthymemes: Body and soul. *Philosophy & Rhetoric*, *5*(4), 201–214.

Olson, C. J. (2014). *Constitutive visions: Indigeneity and commonplaces of national identity in republican Ecuador*. The Pennsylvania State University Press.

Olson, L. C. (2009). Pictorial representations of British America resisting rape: Rhetorical re-circulation of a print series portraying the Boston Port Bill of 1774. *Rhetoric & Public Affairs, 12*(1), 1–35. 10.1353/rap.0.0090

Park, A., Conway, M., & Chen, A. T. (2018). Examining thematic similarity, difference, and membership in three online mental health communities from reddit: A text mining and visualization approach. *Computers in Human Behavior*, *78*, 98–112. 10.1016/j.chb.2017.09.001

Philbin, M. M. (2014). What I got to go through: Normalization and HIV-positive adolescents. *Medical Anthropology, 33*(4), 288–302. 10.1080/01459740.2013.847436

Phillips, W., & Milner, R. M. (2017). *The ambivalent Internet: Mischief, oddity, and antagonism online*. Polity Press.

Přenosil, J. D. (2012). The embodied enthymeme: A hybrid theory of protest. *JAC, 32*(2), 279-303. Retrieved from www.jstor.org/stable/41709683

R/memes. (2020). Reddit. Retrieved February 1, 2020, from https://www.reddit.com/r/memes/.

Rice, J. E. (2008). The new ''new'': Making a case for critical affect studies. *Quarterly Journal of Speech*, *94*(2), 200-212. 10.1080/00335630801975434

Rickert, T.J. (2013). *Ambient rhetoric: The attunements of rhetorical being.* University of Pittsburgh Press.

Riley, S., Rodham, K., & Gavin, J. (2009). Doing weight: Pro-ana and recovery identities in cyberspace. *Journal of Community & Applied Social Psychology*, *19*(5), 348-359. 10.1002/casp.1022

Ruin My Week. (2020, September 7). *Seasonal depression comes and goes, but depression memes are always around (39 Memes)*. https://ruinmyweek.com/memes/depression-memes-list/.

Pratt, R. & Stapelberg, N. J. C. (2018). Early warning biomarkers in major depressive disorder: a strategic approach to a testing question. *Biomarkers, 23*(6), 563-572. 10.1080/1354750X.2018.1463563.

Said, Z. K., & Silbey, J. (2018). Narrative topoi in the digital age. *Journal of Legal Education*, *68*(1), 103–114. Retrieved from papers.ssrn.com/sol3/papers.cfm?abstract_id=3293933

San Jose, A. L., Hall, C. M., Schaefer, B. A., & Breeden, N. C. (2019). How Pinteresting: An analysis of social media resources for internalizing disorders. *Journal of Educational Technology Systems*, *48*(1), 155–185. 10.1177/0047239519828079

Selinger, E., & Hartzog, W. (2016). Facebook's emotional contagion study and the ethical problem of co-opted identity in mediated environments where users lack control. *Research Ethics*, *12*(1), 35–43. https://doi.org/10.1177/1747016115579531

Scott, J. B. (2002). The public policy debate over newborn HIV testing: A case study of the knowledge enthymeme. *Rhetoric Society Quarterly*, *32*(2), 57–83. 10.1080/02773940209391228

Shepherd, R. P. (2020a). What Reddit has to teach us about discourse communities. *Kairos, 24.2*. Retrieved from http://kairos.technorhetoric.net/24.2/praxis/shepherd/index.html

Shepherd, R. P. (2020b). Gaming Reddit's algorithm: r/the_donald, amplification, and the rhetoric of sorting. *Computers and Composition, 56.* Retrieved from https://doi.org/10.1016/j.compcom.2020.102572

Signal-Boost. (2020). *Oxford Dictionary on Lexico.com*. Retrieved from https://www.lexico.com/en/definition/signal-boost.

The Devil's own son? (2020, September 27). *Twitter.* For sale. Baby shoes. Never worn. My wife bought the wrong size and they don't fit our baby, who has big feet. https://twitter.com/stypulkoski/status/1310349471964897280.

Thomas, S. M. (2017). 29 memes that perfectly understood your mental health. *Buzzfeed.* Retrieved from www.buzzfeed.com/soniathomas/29-memes-that-perfectly-understood-your-mental-health

Tiggemann, M., & Zaccardo, M. (2018). "Strong is the new skinny": A content analysis of #fitspiration images on Instagram. *Journal of Health Psychology, 23*(8), 1003–1011. https://doi.org/10.1177/1359105316639436

Twenge, J. M., Gentile, B., DeWall, C. N., Ma, D., Lacefield, K., & Schurtz, D. R. (2010). Birth cohort increases in psychopathology among young Americans, 1938–2007: A cross-temporal meta-analysis of the MMPI. *Clinical Psychology Review, 30*(2), 145-154.

Urban Dictionary: Memes. (2019). Urban Dictionary. Retrieved February 1, 2020, from https://www.urbandictionary.com/define.php?term=Memes

Valdez, A. (2020, September 29). *Twitter.* For sale; baby shoes, never worn, wife didnt think it was funny to try and put on baby shoes on the cat. https://twitter.com/AbrahamValdez_/status/1310847212780433410.

Van Horn, N. M, Beveridge, A., & Morey, S. (2016). Attention ecology: Trend circulation and the virality threshold. *DHQ: Digital Humanities Quarterly, 10*(4), 14–29. Retrieved from http://www.digitalhumanities.org/dhq/vol/10/4/000271/000271.html

Virzi, J. (2019, December 18). *40 memes that might make you laugh if you have crushing depression.* https://www.good.is/articles/memes-about-depression.

Walter, N., Cody, M. J., Xu, L. Z., & Murphy, S. T. (2018). A priest, a rabbi, and a minister walk into a bar: A meta-analysis of humor effects on persuasion. *Human Communication Research*, *44*(4), 343–373. 10.1093/hcr/hqy005

Walton, D. (2001). Enthymemes, common knowledge, and plausible inference. *Philosophy & Rhetoric*, *34*(2), 93-112. 10.1353/par.2001.0010

Wang, J. (2014). Criticising images: Critical discourse analysis of visual semiosis in picture news. *Critical Arts: A South-North Journal of Cultural & Media Studies*, *28*(2), 264–286. 10.1080/02560046.2014.906344

Webb, J. B., Vinoski, E. R., Bonar, A. S., Davies, A. E., & Etzel, L. (2017). Fat is fashionable and fit: A comparative content analysis of Fatspiration and Health at Every Size® Instagram images. *Body Image*, *22*(1), 53–64. 10.1016/j.bodyim.2017.05.003

Wetherbee, B. J. B. (2015). Places in the polity of rhetoric: *Topoi*, evolution, and the fragmentation of discourse. [Doctoral book, Louisville University].

Wickberg, D. (1998). *The senses of humor: Self and laughter in modern America*. Cornell University Press.

WinkGo. (2020, June 16). *61 depression memes that prove laughter is the best medicine*. Retrieved from https://winkgo.com/depression-memes/.

Woods, H. S., & Hahner, L. A. (2019). *Make America meme again: The rhetoric of the alt-right*. Peter Lang Publishing, Inc.

Young, S. L. (2015). Running like a man, sitting like a girl: Visual enthymeme and the case of Caster Semenya. *Women's Studies in Communication, 38*(3), 331–350. 10.1080/07491409.2015.1046623

Zidjaly, N. A. (2017). Memes as reasonably hostile laments: A discourse analysis of political dissent in Oman. *Discourse & Society, 28*(6), 573–594. 10.1177/0957926517721083

Appendix A

WELL, I'VE HIT ROCK BOTTOM, THE ONLY WAY TO GO IS UP!
OH YEAH?!

I'LL SHOW YOU!

realizing you don't feel depressed anymore
realizing you don't feel anything at all anymore

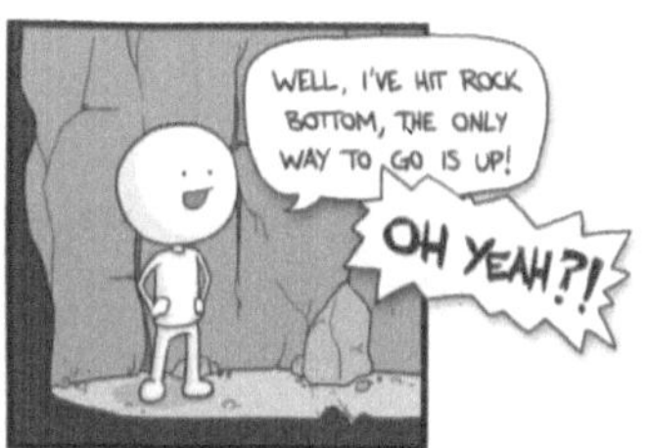

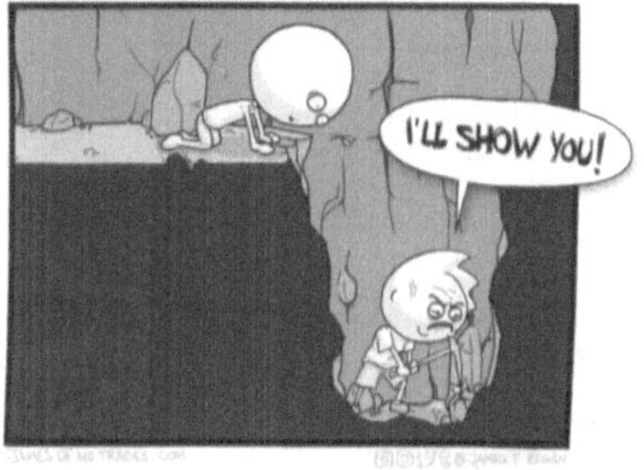

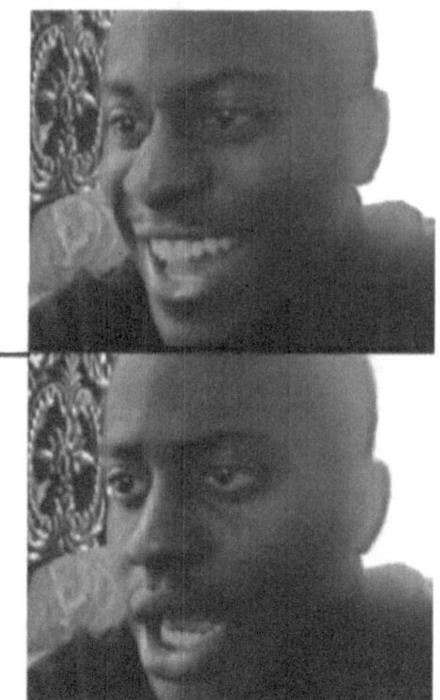

me in my room imagining fake scenarios and hurting my own feelings

antonia
@antoniaella
growing up suicidal is kinda weird cause I didn't think I'd still be alive right now so I don't know what I'm supposed to do with my life or where I'm going because I never planned on being here for it
5/9/18, 5:28 PM
48.8K Retweets 180K Likes

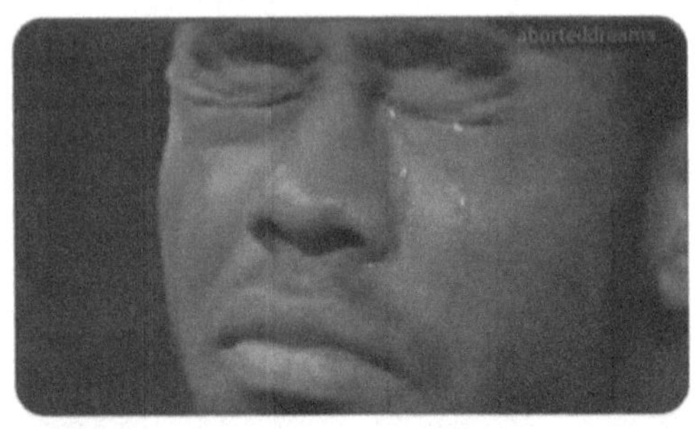

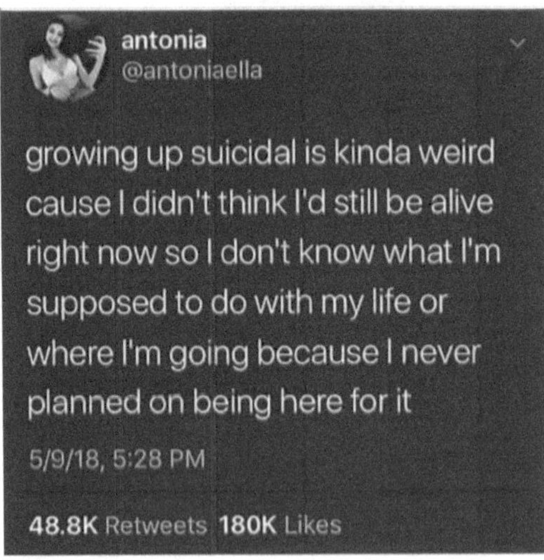

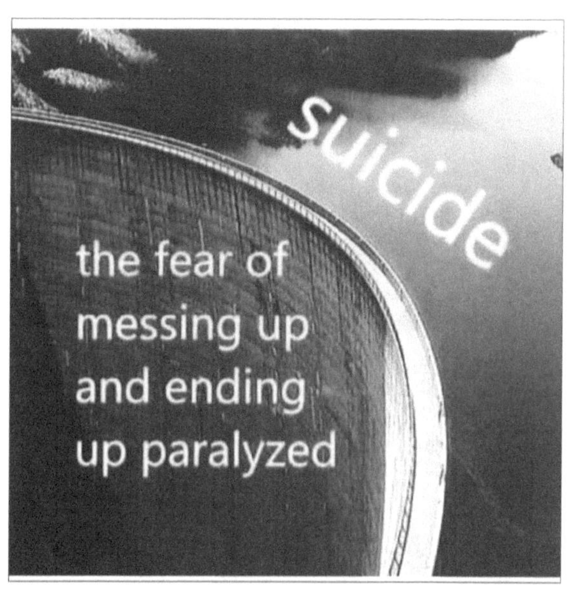
Suicide
the fear of
messing up
and ending
up paralyzed

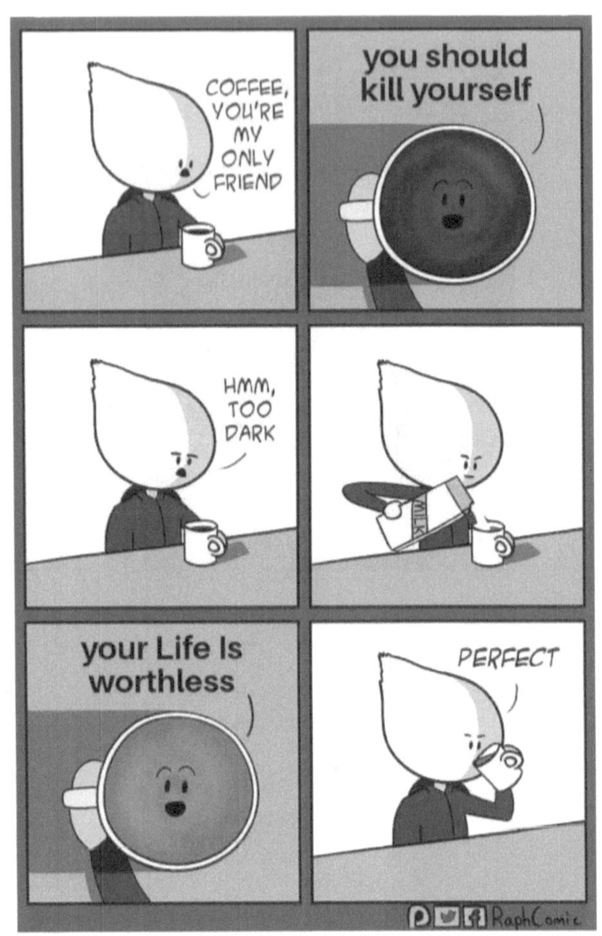
COFFEE, YOU'RE MY ONLY FRIEND
you should kill yourself
HMM, TOO DARK
MILK
your Life Is worthless
PERFECT
RaphComic

When you down a bottle of pills, but wake up in the hospital

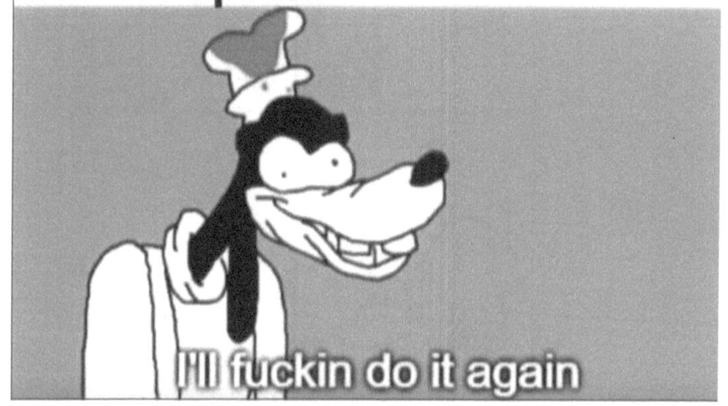

Tsunami:	*T is silent*
Honest:	*H is silent*
Island:	*S is silent*
Queue:	*ueue is silent*
Looking for help:	**everyone goes silent**

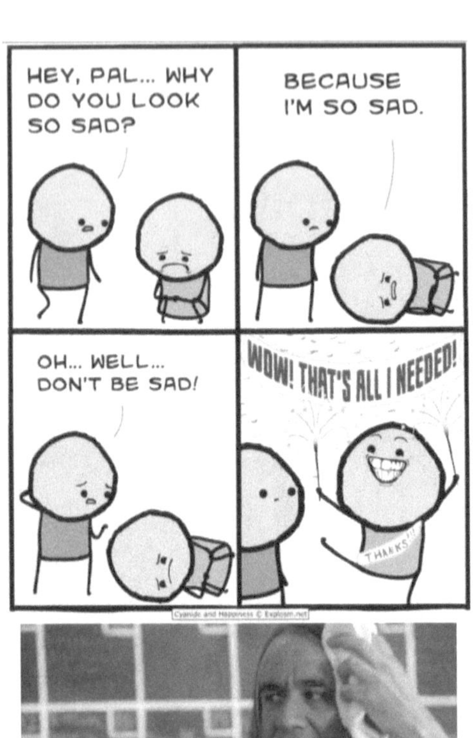
HEY, PAL... WHY DO YOU LOOK SO SAD?
BECAUSE I'M SO SAD.
OH... WELL... DON'T BE SAD!
WOW! THAT'S ALL I NEEDED!
THANKS!!
Cyanide and Happiness © Explosm.net

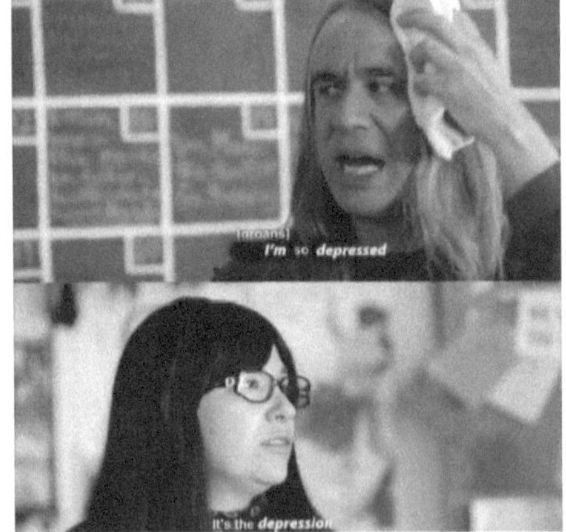
[groans]
I'm so depressed
It's the depression

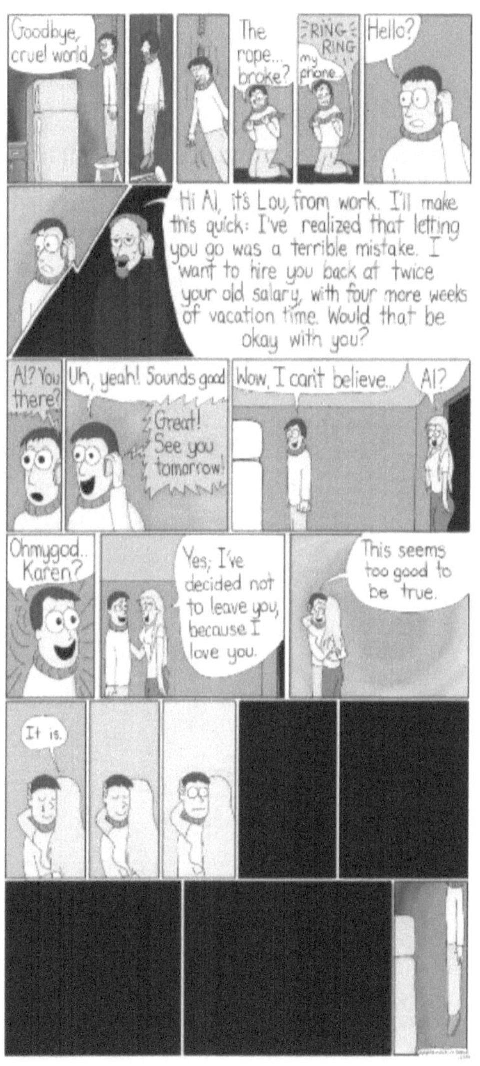

Goodbye, cruel world
The rope... broke?
RING RING
my phone
Hello?
Hi Al, it's Lou, from work. I'll make this quick: I've realized that letting you go was a terrible mistake. I want to hire you back at twice your old salary, with four more weeks of vacation time. Would that be okay with you?
Al? You there?
Uh, yeah! Sounds good
Great! See you tomorrow!
Wow, I can't believe...
Al?
Ohmygod.. Karen?
Yes; I've decided not to leave you, because I love you.
This seems too good to be true.
It is.

Appendix B

Me: *Finally feels a little Happy*

Random suicidal impulse:

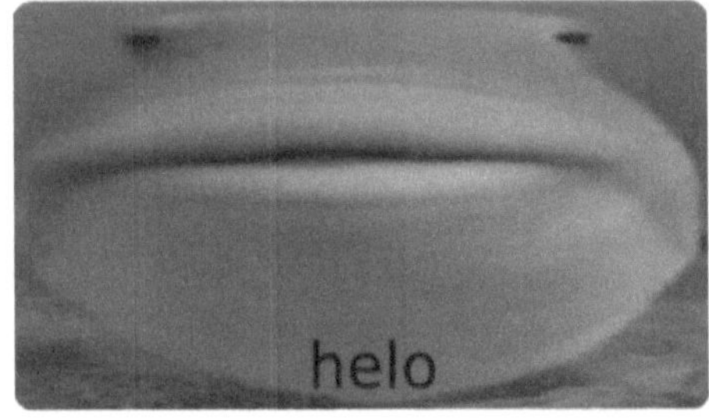

Therapist: and do you think maybe you're choosing to be self destructive?

Me: yup

Therapist: and what are you going to do about that?

Me: probably keep doing it

When you have no interest in being alive but you don't want to hurt your family and friends so instead of killing yourself you just suffer through your existence hoping to be hit by a truck

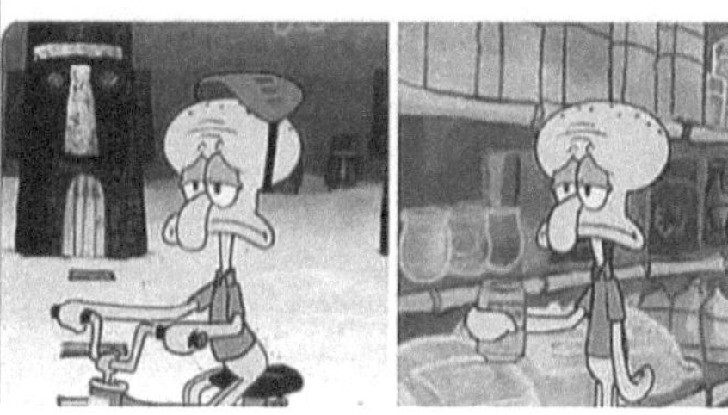

When you find someone who genuinely likes you, finds you attractive and wants to date you

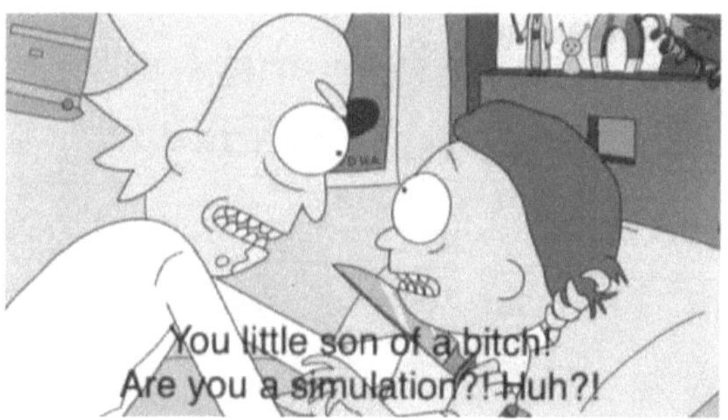

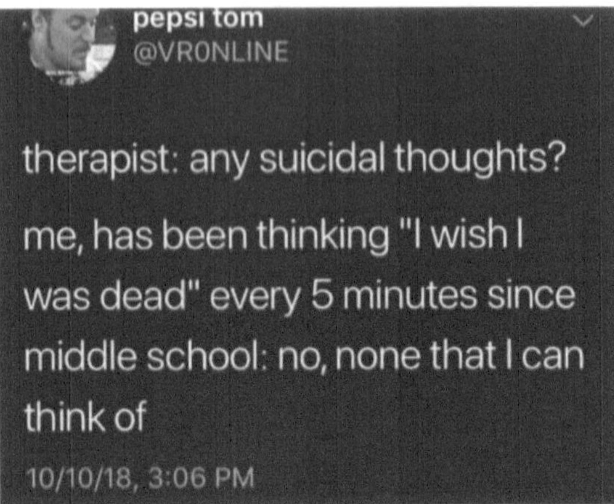

calvin-klein-and-hobbes

How shall I get the Serotonin™ and Dopamine® today??

A. Masturbate

B. Buy myself something I don't need

C. Eat processed food

D. Complete one (1) household task

E. All except D

30,255 notes

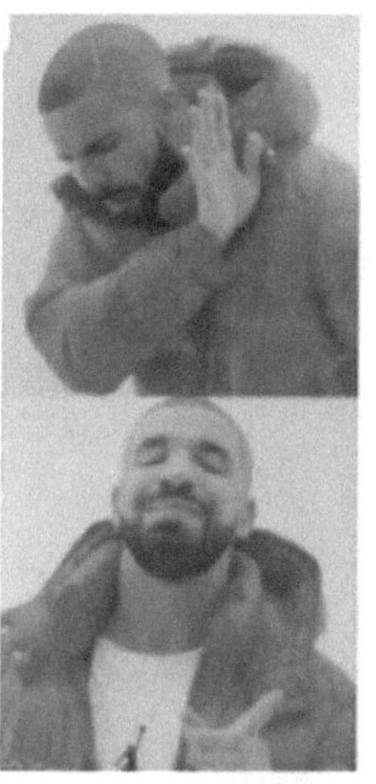
Sharing
our
feelings
Sharing
memes
about how
mentally
fucked up
we are

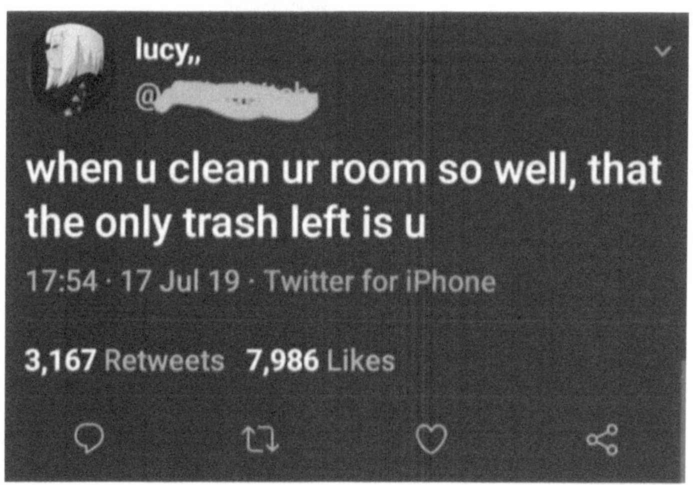
lucy,,
when u clean ur room so well, that the only trash left is u
17:54 · 17 Jul 19 · Twitter for iPhone
3,167 Retweets 7,986 Likes

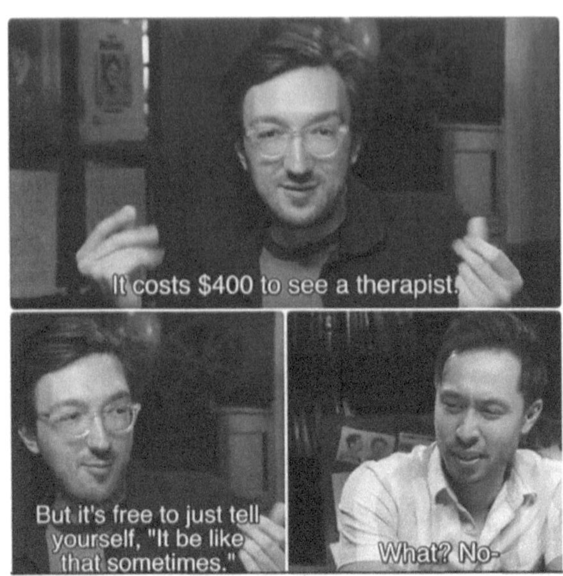
It costs $400 to see a therapist.
But it's free to just tell yourself, "It be like that sometimes."
What? No-

Appendix C

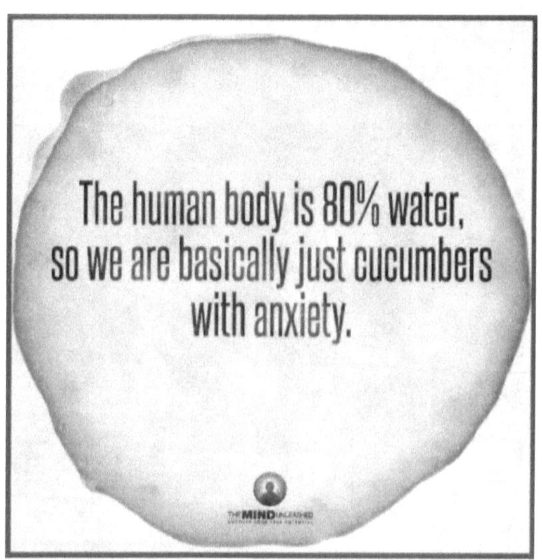

 bluehairedunicorn

Therapist: You're a nice person

Friends: You're a nice person

Family: You're a nice person

Me: Yeah but what if I'm actually shit

 nudityandnerdery

Me: Oh, fuck, I tricked so many people into thinking I'm nice, that's just how shit I am.

thefifthemerald

This post is very loud.

Me giving mental health advice

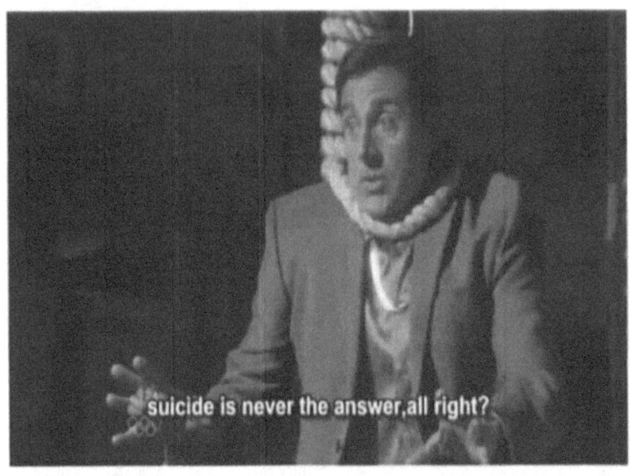

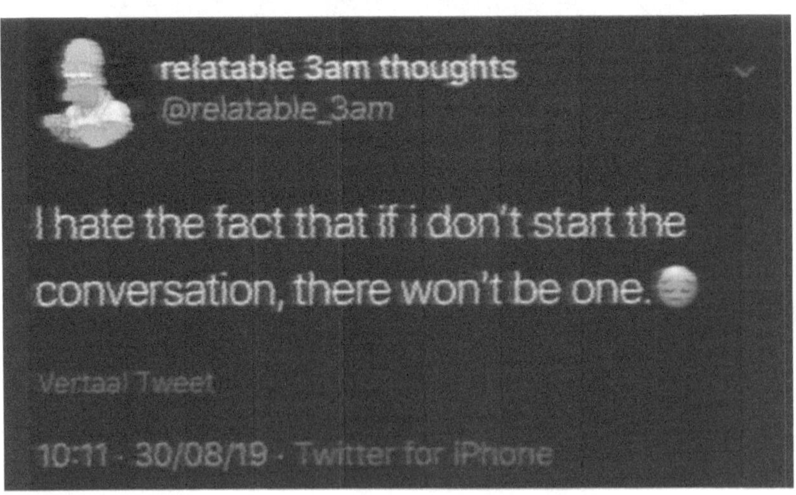

Me, going from socializing with friends to crippling depression in seconds:

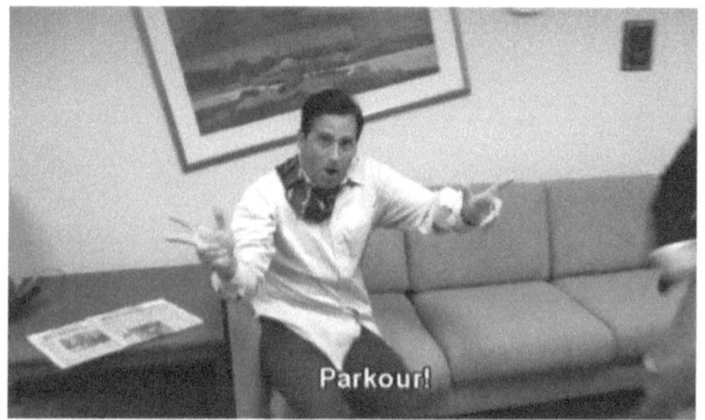

Me when others tell me about their mental health issues:

Me to myself, suffering from mental health issues:

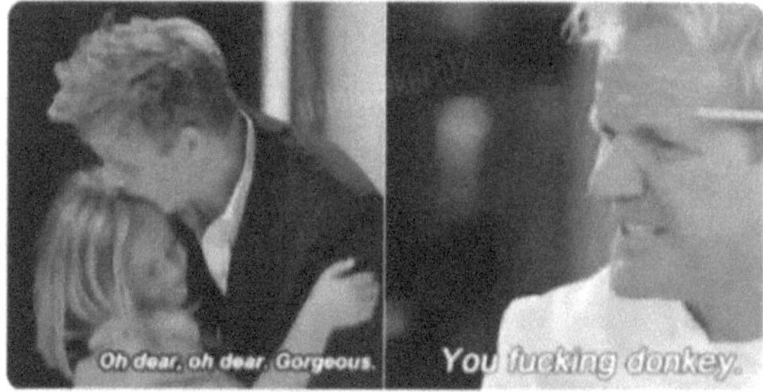

www.ingramcontent.com/pod-product-compliance
Lightning Source LLC
LaVergne TN
LVHW091308150826
845673LV00006B/1576

* 9 7 8 3 3 8 4 2 6 6 8 2 8 *